# Coping with Communication Challenges in Alzheimer's Disease

Marie T. Rau, Ph.D.
Speech-Language Pathologist

SINGULAR PUBLISHING GROUP, INC. Normal
SAN DIEGO, CALIFORNIA
Loan

**Published by Singular Publishing Group, Inc.**
4284 41st Street
San Diego, California 92105-1197

© **1993 by Singular Publishing Group, Inc.**

Typeset in 11/14 Times by CFW Graphics
Printed in the United States of America by BookCrafters

**Library of Congress Cataloging-in-Publication Data**

Rau, Marie T.
    Coping with communication challenges in Alzheimer's disease /
Marie T. Rau.
        p.    cm. — (Coping with aging series)
    Includes index.
    ISBN 1-879105-76-4
    1. Alzheimer's disease—Patients—Care.  2. Communicative
disorders in old age.  I. Title.  II. Series.
RC523.2.R38   1993
618.97′6831—dc20                                     92-41712
                                                          CIP

# ❖ Table of Contents

# ❖ Foreword

The books in the *Coping with Aging Series* are written for men and women coping with the challenges of aging, and for their families and other caregivers. The authors are all experienced practitioners: doctors, nurses, social workers, psychologists, pharmacists, nutritionists, audiologists, physical and occupational therapists, and speech-language pathologists.

The topics of individual volumes are as varied as are the challenges that aging may bring. These include: hearing loss, low vision, depression, sexual dysfunction, immobility, intellectual impairment, language impairment, speech impairment, swallowing impairment, bowel and bladder incontinence, stress of caregiving, giving up independence, medications, and stroke. The volumes themselves, however, share common features. Foremost, they are practical, jargon-free, and responsible. Each contains professionally valid information translated into language people who are not health care providers can understand. Each contains useful advice and sections to help readers decide how they are doing and whether they need to do more, do less, or do something different. Each includes lists of services, suppliers, and additional readings. Each provides evidence that no single person need cope alone.

None of the volumes can substitute for appropriate professional health care. However, when combined with the care, instruction, and counseling that health care providers supply, they make coping with aging easier.

America is greying at the same time its treasury is inadequate to meet its population's needs. Thus the *Coping with Aging Series* offers help for people who need and want to help themselves.

This volume, *Coping with Communication Challenges in Alzheimer's Disease*, is written by a professional speech-language pathologist with more than 25 years of experience in working with adults with communication disorders and with their families. If you, or someone you know, is caring for someone with Alzheimer's disease or a related dementia, this book will be helpful. If you are frustrated or discouraged because your family member is unable to understand what you want him to do or is not able to express himself clearly because of a dementing illness, this book will offer concrete and practical suggestions to help you communicate more effectively. If you are having difficulty meeting some of the other communication challenges faced by the caregiver of a person with dementia, such as communicating with other family members, health care providers, and legal advisers, this book will provide some answers. As you read through this volume, you will see that you and your family member do not need to face the many communication challenges which Alzheimer's disease presents by yourselves.

John C. Rosenbek, Ph.D.
Series Editor

Molly Carnes, M.D.
Medical Editor

# ❖ Preface

This book has been written for family members and others who provide the ongoing, day-to-day care for the estimated 4 million people in the United States who suffer from Alzheimer's disease or related forms of progressive dementia. Despite the persistent myth that present-day families "abandon" their elderly relatives, research has shown that families provide 80 to 90 percent of the ongoing care that frail elderly individuals, including those with dementia, require. Furthermore, families cope while asking relatively little from the formal health care system or government agencies. You, the family caregivers, are the true heroes and heroines in the Alzheimer's disease story. This book, then, is an effort to provide information that will help make your task of caring for a loved one with dementia easier.

Progressive dementia is a devastating disease that eventually affects all aspects of a person's ability to remember, interact, understand, speak, and perform other important tasks of daily living. If the diagnosis of a progressive dementia has been confirmed, you, the family caregiver, will need to begin to plan to deal with these changes, including communication changes, as they occur.

The theme of the book is communication — communication between the person with Alzheimer's disease and his or her caregivers, between family members and health care professionals, between and among concerned family members and friends. Most of the issues and problems that arise in the daily care of the person with dementia involve communication in one way or another. It is hoped that if the importance of communication is understood, and suggestions for dealing with the communication difficulties that occur are offered, you'll be able to cope more effectively and successfully.

## Overview

Because the focus of this book is on communication, Chapter 1 defines and describes what communication involves, and the purposes communication serves in human interactions. The importance of effective communication is stressed. The chapter also presents information about changes and stability in communication abilities as part of the normal process of aging. Chapter 2 provides basic information about the dementias, especially Alzheimer's disease, the most frequently occurring dementing illness. A discussion of the nature of communication problems in dementia follows.

Chapters 3, 4, and 5 provide more detail about the general patterns of communication difficulty observed in what have been described as the phases, or stages, of progressive dementing illness: early (mild), middle (moderate), and late (severe).

In Chapter 6, some general principles and guidelines for enhancing communication with the person with dementia are discussed. These principles can be applied at any phase of the disease. Chapters 7, 8, and 9 describe specific strategies for dealing with communication difficulties and sustaining communication with your family member in the early, middle, and late stages of the illness.

Alzheimer's disease and other progressive dementias can take their toll not only on the primary caregiver, but on family relationships as well. Chapter 10 deals with communication between and among family members in caring for the person with dementia. Of special importance is the caregiver's ability to be able to communicate the need for assistance in meeting the increasingly greater needs of the family member with dementia. How to ask for help and accept help when offered are crucial survival strategies. Chapter 11 discusses other sources of assistance and opportunities for communication, including caregiver support groups.

As the caregiver of someone with Alzheimer's disease you must also communicate with a variety of professionals: physicians, nurses, other health care providers; lawyers; and representatives of governmental and private service agencies. Suggestions for successfully advocating for your family member and for yourself in these interactions are found in Chapters 12, 13, and 14. Chapter 15 discusses the relationship between some of the common behavior changes seen in people with Alzheimer's disease and communication difficulties. Following a concluding chapter (Chapter 16), a listing of some useful supplemental resources are contained in Chapter 17. Finally, a glossary of terms related to dementing illness is found in the Appendix.

## A Word About Inclusive Language

It is difficult to know which gender to use when speaking or writing about dementia. The "typical" person with dementia of the Alzheimer's type is an elderly woman, being cared for by her daughter or daughter-in-law. On the other hand, the population with whom I work is almost exclusively male, and their caregivers female, usually spouses or daughters. For the sake of less awkward and cumbersome prose, I have arbitrarily chosen to use the male personal pronoun forms to stand for both male and female when referring to the person with dementia.

# ❖ Acknowledgment

A special note of thanks to Gordon Campbell, R.N., a nurse practitioner who works with people with dementia and with their caregivers on a daily basis. He provided valuable insights and suggestions regarding what caregivers want and need to know.

For John and Betty

# Chapter 1

# Communication

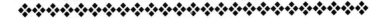

When an injury, illness, or disease (such as Alzheimer's disease) disrupts the brain's ability to take in and remember information, one of the functions that is affected is the ability to communicate effectively with one's family and friends. Feelings of frustration, anger, and helplessness may surface because the individual is unable to remember the name of a familiar object or a well-known person. Family members, too, feel helpless and frustrated when they are not able to interpret their loved one's communications or when the affected family member misunderstands them.

## What is Communication?

To understand what happens when communication is disrupted by disease or by damage to the brain, we need to explore first what is involved in normal human communication. "Communication" is a broad term that includes all of the ways in which people send and receive messages. Speaking, listening, reading, writing, and gesturing or pantomime are all forms of communication. Drawing, sign language, facial expression, and body postures are other forms of communication between and among people.

Some of these types of communication involve *sending* messages (speaking, writing, pantomiming) and others involve *receiving* messages (listening; reading; and "reading" someone's facial expression, tone of voice, or body posture). For communication to occur, there must be at least one sender and one receiver of a message. In our everyday lives, we continually switch roles as senders and receivers of messages.

## How are Speech and Language Different?

It's important to distinguish between two components of the human communication system, that is, between *speech* and *language*. Different brain diseases, including Alzheimer's disease, can affect different aspects of communication. For us to understand *why* someone is having difficulty communicating, and *what* might be done to help them communicate more effectively, we need to know whether speech, or language, or both are affected. Some conditions, such as a stroke affecting the nerves that control the muscles of the tongue and/or larynx (voice box), will disturb speech, but not language. Alzheimer's disease, on the other hand, can affect some aspects of language functioning early, while leaving the person's ability to speak intact until later in the disease. Let's explore this distinction in more detail.

*Speech* refers to the vocal expression of words or thoughts through the use of the lungs, vocal cords, mouth cavity, tongue, lips, and teeth to produce sounds that others can understand. Speech production, in other words, deals with the *mechanics* of combining sounds into words and sentences. Hundreds of finely controlled and rapidly occurring muscle movements are involved in speaking even a single sentence — a skill mastered by most speakers of a language by the age of 4 or 5!

The term *language* refers to both the vocabulary, or dictionary, of individual words through which people share meanings (called *semantics*) as well as the ways in which they change words or put words together in a certain order to express different thoughts (called *syntax*). "The man bit the dog" means something quite different from "the dog bit the man." "The girl wrote a letter" means something different from "The girls wrote a letter." As a person learns his native language, he attaches meaning to more and more words, while at the same time he is learning to combine words into meaningful sentences. Language, then, is a shared set of symbols and the rules for changing or combining those symbols to express thoughts and ideas. Language can be spoken, written, pictured, or gestured.

## Nonverbal Communication

We communicate a great deal of information through facial expression, body posture, and tone of voice. When someone is feeling sad or depressed, this may be signaled by a sad facial expression, drooping shoulders, and a "depressed" voice quality, rather than by spoken words. At times, the words that we say may not "match" our tone of voice or the expression on our face. For example, we may communicate anger or boredom through facial expression and voice, while the words that we say may be polite and positive. When this happens, the listener is more likely to pay attention to the angry or bored expression and vocal tone than to the words themselves.

Gestures also communicate a great deal of information to another person. A gentle touch, a hug, a reassuring pat on the back can convey a positive message to the communication partner. At the same time, a gesture of rejection, disgust, or anger sends a negative message that is stronger than any accompanying words. This nonverbal communication is extremely important in the total process of sending and receiving information. As we shall discuss in later chapters, nonverbal messages can be a reassuring link to the person with dementia who has difficulty understanding speech and expressing himself verbally. The capacity to understand nonverbal messages, such as touch, tone of voice, and gesture, may remain intact when verbal comprehension and expression is no longer working well.

## The Pragmatics of Communication

Other important features of communication exchanges involve what is called the *pragmatics* of communication. Pragmatics is the study of the ways in which people *use* communication: for example, to ask questions, to explain an idea, to make a request, to argue or demand. People who study pragmatics are interested in the purposes and intentions behind our spoken words or gestures. Pragmatics also involves what human communicators know about the "rules" of conversation: turn taking, listening when someone else is speaking, and maintaining eye contact with the person with whom you're speaking, for example. We've all experienced how annoying it can be when we're involved in a conversation with someone who breaks these rules and interrupts us or looks away when we're talking to them.

When illness or injury disrupts brain function, one or more of these important features of communication (speech, language, nonverbal communication, pragmatics) may be affected. In Chapter 2 we will explore how progressive dementing illness can profoundly disrupt some aspects of communication and leave others relatively intact until the late stages of the disease.

## Normal Aging and Communication: What Can We Expect?

It is a common experience for middle aged and older people to wonder if they are "losing" their memory or "getting senile" when they have some difficulty remembering an acquaintance's name or coming up with a specific word. Most of us over the age of 40 have had such concerns and thoughts at times. We may ask ourselves, "Is this the beginning of Alzheimer's disease? Will this 'forgetting' get worse?" We may be especially concerned if there is a history of dementing illness in the family. On the other hand, it is not uncommon for family members to ignore the warning signs that something is truly wrong with the memory, thinking, and communication functions of an older family member suffering from early dementing illness. They explain away these changes as signs of normal aging: "After all, Grandma is almost eighty. What can we expect!"

For a better understanding of the communication difficulties related to dementia, it is important to appreciate the distinction between the early signs and symptoms of this progressive *illness* and normal, age-related changes in memory and word recall. There are clear differences between the changes in memory, thinking, and communication that are a normal part of aging and the declines in these abilities that are part of the illness called Alzheimer's disease. Dementia is not normal at any age! In the rest of this chapter you will learn about cognitive and communication changes that are part of the normal aging process, in contrast to dementia.

## Changes in Memory and Thinking

It is more accurate to speak of human memory capacities as "memories" in the plural, rather than "memory" in the singular, for it is now known and understood that we use several different types of memories. Memory capacities can be described in relation to *time* (immediate, short-term, long-term) or in terms of *what* is remembered (a particular event, what something means, how a task is performed). Some of these memory functions will be relatively undisturbed by the aging process, while others may be diminished somewhat by the physical changes that are a part of growing older (*age-related changes*). In the following discussion, what happens to memory functions in the normal course of growing older will be contrasted with the effects on memory functions of dementing illnesses, such as Alzheimer's disease.

### Immediate Memory

We have a capacity known as "immediate memory," which allows us to remember a telephone number, or to repeat a sentence just as we heard it. Generally, we do not store these kinds of memories for more than a few seconds — just long enough to use them and "forget" them. The normal human immediate memory capacity is about seven numbers or other "bits" of information. Our immediate memory capacities remain intact during the process of normal aging. In the course of a progressive dementing illness, immediate memory abilities will also remain intact until the late stages of the disease.

### Short-Term Memory

In addition to this immediate memory, we also are able to store items in memory for relatively short periods of time, that is, for minutes to a few days. We can usually remember without difficulty what we had for dinner the night before, or who stopped by for a visit last Sunday afternoon. Short-term memory is very important to daily life and to being able to function independently. It assists us in remembering what daily tasks need to be done, what phone calls we need to return, and that lunch date we've made. Short-term memory helps us remember that we've driven to the store for milk, rather than eggs. In the course of normal aging, we retain functional short-term memory ability, while in dementing illness short-term memory is eventually severely affected.

## Long-Term Memory

For a person to be able to remember information for longer periods of time, it must first be stored in short-term memory where it can be "rehearsed." Most of us have had the experience of trying to remember a good joke long enough to share it with someone else. We make an effort to remember the joke, perhaps rehearsing it to ourselves, so that we can retell it at an appropriate moment.

Information that we store in what is called long-term memory is available to be retrieved when needed: our address, telephone number, or social security number, for example. Our ability to recognize familiar places and faces, or information we learned long ago, also calls on long-term memory. In the course of normal aging, most people will notice that they don't remember names or details as efficiently as when they were younger. Relevant and important long-term memories, however, will not be lost.

## Episodic Memory

Memory for specific events that have occurred in our experience is called "episodic" memory, that is, we consciously recollect details of episodes in our lives that happened in a particular time and place. We might remember, for example, the details of a delicious dinner we ate at a favorite restaurant last week — what we had to eat, who was with us, the general atmosphere, and so forth. Episodic memory requires remembering *what, when, with whom,* and often *where.* Episodic memory involves information from both short-term and long-term memory, that is, memories related to events that happened from a few moments ago to a long time in the past.

Healthy older individuals do experience some difficulty with episodic memory. We may not remember things that have happened in the recent past quite as well or as quickly as we did when we were younger. This loss of efficiency in the working of episodic memory is sometimes referred to as "benign forgetfulness" or "age-associated memory impairment" (AAMI). The healthy elderly adult may, for example, forget some details of a past experience, but not the whole experience. Normally aging people will usually remember forgotten details at a later time (or when more relaxed) and are usually able to use notes and other reminders to aid episodic memory.

In contrast, failure of episodic memory is a major, defining symptom of progressive dementia. The person with Alzheimer's disease will forget whole experiences, even those that have occurred only moments before. He will rarely remember these experiences later and will gradually be unable to use memory aids. Impairment of episodic memory will eventually lead to the person with Alzheimer's disease being unable to care for himself. Inability to function in daily life because of memory loss is *not* a characteristic of age-related memory impairment.

**Semantic Memory**

Besides specific events and their details, we have a more general memory capacity — for the meanings of words and the concepts or ideas that those words represent. This type of memory, called "semantic memory," is what enables us to understand other speakers, follow directions, and respond to requests. Answers to questions such as, "What do you use a fork for?" and "Who was Babe Ruth?" are retrieved from semantic memory.

What happens to this memory function as we age? As we grow older, it is true that our brains become less efficient at coming up with specific words when we want them. We more frequently experience what has been called the "tip of the tongue" phenomenon. You have probably heard people say, "I can't remember that fellow's name, but its right on the tip of my tongue. I think it starts with a 'b'!" Nevertheless, memory for the *meanings* of words and related concepts remains intact as we age. In fact, our vocabulary, or the dictionary of word meanings stored in our brain, continues to grow throughout our lifetime. Healthy older people likewise don't usually have difficulty remembering the names of familiar items or well-known people.

In Alzheimer's disease, on the other hand, semantic memory as well as episodic memory is diminished. Recent research suggests that, in Alzheimer's disease, problems with semantic memory may, at least at first, be due to impaired *access* to what is stored in semantic memory, rather than to loss of the concepts or word meanings themselves. For example, the person affected by Alzheimer's disease may be able to show that he knows what the word "table" means when he is given a cue such as "Which one would you put your dishes on?" or when the task is simple enough for him to understand what is being asked of him. As time passes, however, loss of semantic memory capacity will eventually make it difficult for the person with dementia to understand and follow written or spoken directions and requests.

### Procedural Memory

When we sit down at a piano to play a familiar tune or type out a letter on a computer or typewriter keyboard, we are utilizing *procedural memory*. Likewise, when we climb onto a bicycle or a pair of skis, we "remember" how to use them. Procedural memory is considered the most basic type of memory. It simply requires a person to perform a previously experienced activity. Procedural memory does not require *conscious* recollection on our part, but does show that we have previously had a particular experience. Current evidence suggests that this type of memory is not affected by normal aging, and that it is largely spared in Alzheimer's disease as well, at least until the later stages.

### Thinking Abilities

Our ability to think (to learn, to exercise judgment, to act reasonably) is, of course, related to the ability to remember in the first place. Thinking abilities, especially for learning new information, slow down a bit as we age. A normal older person can learn some types of new material as well as a younger person, but not as quickly. On the other hand, judgment and reasoning abilities remain sound in the healthy older person, even into very old age. In Alzheimer's disease, the ability to learn new information, to think logically, and to use good judgment will gradually be lost.

## Speech and Language Functions

Other than the mild, occasional word recall problems mentioned previously, language abilities remain intact in the normal course of aging. The ability to associate words and their meanings and to combine words to express what we mean is unchanged. Knowledge of the "rules" of social communication is not diminished. Healthy elders remain, all in all, good communicators!

The body structures we use for speaking, such as the lungs, larynx (voice box), tongue, lips, and palate (soft part of the roof of the mouth) undergo some physical changes with age, as do all body structures. These changes, however, are not significant nor do they usually interfere with daily communication in healthy older individuals. Even for relatively healthy elders, however, lack of teeth or ill-fitting dentures can contribute to making speech less clear. Poor hearing, a common problem in the elderly, makes communication more difficult. Visual problems can interfere with the older person's ability to understand facial expression, gestures, and written communication. For any older person, problems with vision, hearing, or dentures need attention so that communication skills are maintained.

Speech and language changes seen in dementing illness will be described in upcoming chapters (especially Chapters 3, 4, and 5) and so will not be dealt with here.

## Personality Factors

We often use the word "personality" in describing people and how they appear or "seem" to us. We might, for example, say "He has a pleasant personality," "John has a hard-driving personality," or "She has a difficult personality" in relating our overall impression of a person.

The way individuals view the world, deal with stresses, and interact with other people all appear to be factors that go into making up their "personality." At times we may describe someone's personality based on how comfortable we feel when we're with that person (for example, "She's a tense person" or "She has an easy going personality").

Do people change in basic outlook and the way they cope with challenges as they grow older? Studies that have looked over time at individuals' attitudes and ways of managing their lives suggest that significant personality changes *do not* take place as one grows older. Some people may become slightly more socially withdrawn in old age; however, this may be due to changes in their living situation and health circumstances, rather than to changes in basic personality. Although some older individuals may become "more emphatically themselves" as certain personality traits become emphasized in old age, research suggests that human beings maintain consistency of personality throughout their adult lives.

Major personality changes in an older person may be an indication of a condition (such as depression or dementia) that needs medical evaluation. Chapter 2 provides an overview of dementing illness, focusing especially on Alzheimer's disease. Symptoms of this disease, including personality changes, are discussed in more detail in Chapter 2.

# Chapter 2

# Dementia

Over the last 10 years, U.S. society has given increasing attention and resources to the study of Alzheimer's disease and other dementias. Why has this occurred? A major reason can be found if we look at some numbers. Currently, about 4 million Americans are afflicted with dementia (Aronson, 1988). Because of the aging of our population, that number is expected to triple over the next 50 years (Cohen & Eisdorfer, 1986). Of this number, more than half will be victims of Alzheimer's disease, the most common type of dementia (Aronson, 1988). Although some younger individuals (people in their 40s and 50s) are victims of Alzheimer's disease, it is primarily a disease of the elderly. Between 4 and 5 percent of the population over age 65 is described as having a severe dementia (Mortimer, Schuman, & French, 1986). At age 80, a person's chances of developing a severe dementia increase to about 20 percent, or one in five. (Aronson, 1988). Dementia is the fourth leading cause of death among the elderly in the United States (Powell & Courtice, 1983). As the number of older people in our society increases, especially the number over the age of 75, the need for continued research into the causes of and possible treatments for dementing illnesses has grown more urgent.

# What is Dementia?

Dementia is a general term indicating brain failure in older individuals. It is not a disease as such, but rather a group of *symptoms* that indicate the need for further medical evaluation. These symptoms can include: gradual loss of short-term memory (the ability to remember what occurred minutes to days before); loss of other intellectual abilities; and changes in behavior, mood, and personality. Communication abilities, especially language skills, may also show early signs of deterioration. There are a number of medical conditions and diseases that can result in the group of symptoms we call "dementia." The two most common, Alzheimer's disease and multi-infarct dementia, are discussed below.

## Alzheimer's Disease

The most common form of dementia is Alzheimer's disease, an irreversible, usually slowly progressive illness affecting memory, learning ability, judgment, language, emotional expression, behavior, and personality. This disease accounts for slightly more than half of the diagnosed cases of dementia in the United States.

Alzheimer's disease was named after a German pathologist, Dr. Alois Alzheimer, who first described the condition in 1906. It is a diagnosis that can only be made with certainty at autopsy, when the brain tissue of someone suspected of having the disease can be examined. The brain tissue of people with Alzheimer's disease shows characteristic patterns that confirm the diagnosis. In Alzheimer's disease, groups of nerve endings in the brain's outer layer (the cortex) die, disrupting the transmission between nerve cells of important brain electrochemical signals. These clusters of degenerated nerve cells are called *plaques*. Changes also occur in the nerve cells of the cortex. This causes a buildup of abnormal fibers called *neurofibrillary tangles.* A certain number of these plaques and tangles have been found in the brains of older people who showed no signs of dementia while living; however, they are found in much greater numbers in the brains of people who had been diagnosed in life as having Alzheimer's disease. Researchers have found a relationship between the number of plaques and tangles observed in brain tissue and the severity of memory loss and intellectual decline observed while the person was alive. Because the diagnosis cannot be confirmed except at autopsy, some people prefer to use the term "Dementia of the Alzheimer's Type" (DAT).

In addition to being a clinical, or probable diagnosis during a person's lifetime, dementia of the Alzheimer's type is also a "diagnosis of exclusion." That is, when all other possible causes for a pattern of general deterioration of memory, cognitive, and social/emotional functions have been ruled out, a diagnosis of Alzheimer's disease is likely. This method of diagnosing Alzheimer's disease by exclusion has been found to be 80 to 90 percent accurate.

## Multi-Infarct Dementia

About 20 percent of dementia cases result from the person having suffered many small strokes over a period of time (Aronson, 1988). This form of dementia is called *multi-infarct dementia,* or MID. Symptoms of multi-infarct disease will vary, depending on the areas of the brain affected. For example, speech and language functions may be more affected than other abilities. Individuals with multi-infarct dementia sometimes show a "stair-step" pattern of brain failure, with further declines in function noted after new stroke events. Other people with this type of dementia may show more gradual and steady loss of abilities over time.

Multi-infarct dementia is, to some extent, treatable, although the damage already done to brain cells by strokes cannot be reversed. If the occurrence of small strokes is diagnosed early, likely causes such as high blood pressure can be treated with medication. The prevention of strokes is an important reason for treating high blood pressure and other conditions such as diabetes as early as possible. Cigarette smoking is another major contributing factor in putting someone at risk for strokes.

## Mixed Dementia

Some individuals (about 25 percent of dementia victims) have a combination of Alzheimer's disease and multi-infarct dementia. Taken together, Alzheimer's disease and stroke-related dementias account for 90 percent of dementia cases.

# Treatable or Reversible Causes of Dementia

Other conditions, including medically treatable ones, that can look like progressive dementia in its early stages include depression; hormone deficiency (especially chronic, severe low thyroid hormone levels); and increased pressure on the brain from bleeding, brain tumors, or a blocking of the flow of brain fluid (cerebrospinal fluid) causing a condition called hydrocephalus. The improper use of drugs, especially sleeping pills and alcohol, can also cause a person to show signs of dementia. If your family member is showing behaviors suggestive of a dementia, but a diagnosis of an irreversible dementia has not been made, a medical evaluation, including an evaluation by a physician who specializes in diagnosing and treating brain dysfunction (a neurologist), is in order. Some of the conditions just mentioned may be at least partially reversible.

## Focus on Alzheimer's Disease

Because it is the most common form of dementing illness, the remainder of this book will focus on Alzheimer's disease. The descriptions of communication decline outlined in Chapters 3, 4, and 5, for example, reflect behaviors typically seen in people with Alzheimer's disease. Nevertheless, many of the suggestions offered for enhancing communication can be used with people who have other forms of dementia. The terms "Alzheimer's disease," "dementia of the Alzheimer's type," and "dementia" will be used interchangeably throughout the book to refer to dementia of the Alzheimer's type.

## The Stages of Alzheimer's Disease

Because Alzheimer's disease is characterized usually by a gradual onset and slow, steady declines in a variety of functions over time, it does not have clearly defined stages or phases. Furthermore, people with dementia will show varying *rates* of decline. Some people may stay at a plateau in their illness for several years, while other individuals (especially those afflicted at younger ages) may decline more rapidly. There will also be some variation from person to person in the rate at which certain skills deteriorate compared to other abilities. People with Alzheimer's disease may show inconsistent ability to accomplish certain tasks from day to day as well, although the progress of the disease overall is a gradual decline in these abilities.

Despite the difficulties in attempting to describe clearly defined stages of the illness, people have found it useful to use the terms "mild," "moderate," and "severe" to indicate the broad and overlapping phases of Alzheimer's disease. We will use this same somewhat loose definition of stages in describing the decline in communication abilities seen in dementia of the Alzheimer's type.

## Symptoms of Alzheimer's Disease: An Overview

Alzheimer's disease, as has been stated, will result in changes in memory functions, personality, behavior, and, in the later stages, physical functions. A brief description of the changes seen in each of these areas follows.

## Changes in Memory

In the early stages, the disease will affect certain types of memory more than others. Short-term memory, that is, memory for things that have happened from a few minutes ago to a few days ago, will be affected first. Deterioration of this short-term memory is responsible for the repetitious questions and statements characteristic of Alzheimer's disease. Memory for the meaning of words and ideas (semantic memory) will gradually be affected, resulting in reduced vocabulary and problems with understanding verbal messages.

In the late stages of the disease, even memories for events and people from the distant past (long-term memory) will become fragmentary. While increased forgetfulness is often seen as "normal" for older people, it will gradually become obvious that something is wrong as the person gets lost in unfamiliar places, forgets basic safety precautions around the house (such as turning off the stove), or fails to recognize and remember the names of familiar acquaintances. Other common warning signs are failing ability to keep a checkbook or to perform familiar work tasks.

## Personality Changes

Families often report that personality changes in their relative were the first clues they had that "something was wrong." Early changes in personality thought to be related to the Alzheimer's disease process have been described as "apathy," or a "flattening" of the personality and emotions, giving the impression that the person "doesn't care." The affected person may gradually lose interest in previously enjoyed activities, including reading, sports, or card games. He may show less drive and have trouble getting tasks started. He may overreact to certain situations in untypical ways, or seem more irritable than usual.

## Depression

At the same time, some of these early personality changes may be the individual's reaction to what he is experiencing as memory fails him and once simple tasks become perplexing and difficult. The possibility that the person with mild dementia is depressed needs to be considered. Feelings of depression are not uncommon in the early stages of Alzheimer's disease. What's important to know is that, while there is currently no known cure or medical treatment for Alzheimer's disease, the depression that often accompanies early dementing illness may respond well to medical treatment. If depression goes untreated, it can result in a lower level of functioning, or what has been called "excess disability" in dementia. Chapter 15 offers suggestions for dealing with depression.

## Behavior Changes

The behavior symptoms of Alzheimer's disease can include, in the early stages, irritability, denial that anything is wrong, overreacting, and repetitive questions. In the later phases of the illness, wakefulness at night, restlessness or pacing, wandering, hostility, suspiciousness, unsafe actions, refusal to cooperate in basic care tasks such as bathing, and problems with eating are some of the behaviors that may be distressing to you as a caregiver. Keep in mind, however, that all people with dementia do not exhibit all of these behaviors. Hostile and physically aggressive behaviors, in particular, tend to be rare. In Chapter 15, some of the more common "problem behaviors" are discussed, and their possible links to communication deficits are examined. Also in Chapter 15, you'll find ideas for coping with troublesome behaviors. Specific suggestions for dealing with difficult behaviors can be found in many of the references listed in Chapter 17 as well.

## Tolerance for Stress

Most of us can handle the stresses of living busy lives quite well, at least most of the time. We can answer the telephone, referee a fight between the children, and keep an eye on the stove at the same time, for example. At work, we may be able to deal with several tasks in the course of a day, going from one to the other without becoming upset or losing our working rhythm. We can concentrate on the task at hand in the midst of background noise and remember the next thing that we need to do. For the person with Alzheimer's disease, though, the ability to deal with what seem like normal stresses decreases. As the disease worsens, the person's "stress threshold" is lowered, and he becomes less able to deal with all of the information and stimulation around him. His brain can no longer handle this "overload."

## Good Days and Bad Days

At the same time, the person with dementia will typically show an inconsistent pattern in his ability to complete tasks or to understand and communicate. In the early and middle stages of the disease, he may have "good days and bad days." This can be very confusing to you as the caregiver. You may think, because he did well yesterday and is unable to function at that same level today, that he is "being stubborn," or just "being difficult." On the other hand, if he has a few good days in a row, the temptation is to hope that somehow the disease process has slowed, or that your relative is "getting better." It's important to keep in mind when you see these fluctuations in abilities in your family member that they are very likely *not under his control,* but rather a characteristic of the disease itself.

## But He *Looks* So Good!

One of the most difficult things for family members and friends to deal with is the discrepancy between the *physical appearance* of the person with mild-to-moderate Alzheimer's disease, and his *declining mental abilities.* We expect someone with a disease to look ill! When we see a healthy appearing, physically strong person who can't remember his children's names, and who gets lost in his familiar neighborhood, it doesn't make sense. In some respects, Alzheimer's is a "hidden" disease because the affected person doesn't appear to have anything wrong with him. People with dementia and their caregivers need help and support to deal with the lack of understanding and sympathy they may feel at times from people who don't know about dementing illness.

## Physical Functioning

Typically, physical problems will not be observed in the early and into the middle stages of Alzheimer's disease. Later, your relative may develop difficulty in walking, as well as in activities such as dressing, grooming, bathing, and eating. For example, your relative may be unable to remember *how* to complete such a seemingly simple activity as brushing his teeth. Such activities require that the brain be able to *plan* the muscle movements necessary to complete them, even without the person thinking about what he is doing (after all, we don't usually think about how we are walking, or what we need to do to bring the fork to our mouth).

Eventually, in the final stages, the person with progressive dementia may lose control over bladder and bowels (incontinence) and swallowing ability and become quite physically dependent, even bedridden.

## Communication

Just as early memory problems may be almost imperceptible, the first stages of communication loss in Alzheimer's disease may resemble the occasional difficulties many older people experience in coming up with specific words. Gradually, however, problems in finding the right word will become more obvious, and speech will begin to sound more "empty." For example, words such as "thing" and "stuff" will substitute for the specific names of items such as "fork" and "dishes." Thoughts will become harder to express and gradually become less coherent. The ability to understand verbal messages will decline and there will be less initiation of conversation. When the disease has become severe, only repetitious sounds, words, or phrases may be heard, or little speech at all. Usually, communication decline will be consistent with the rate and amount of memory loss and the loss of other brain functions.

# The Causes of Alzheimer's Disease

We do not know the actual cause or causes of Alzheimer's disease. Research is ongoing, and some promising discoveries have recently been made related to possible virus causes, immune system deficiencies, and disturbances in the production of certain brain chemical "messengers," in particular one called *acetylcholine.* It is known, for example, that the amount of acetylcholine is significantly reduced in Alzheimer's disease, but the reason for this is not known. In rare families, where many members have Alzheimer's disease, genetics or heredity may play a role. Usually though, Alzheimer's disease only affects a single member of a family.

## The Role of Aluminum

There has been quite a bit of attention focused on the role of the metal aluminum as a possible cause of Alzheimer's disease. Many caregivers have questions such as, "Should

I get rid of my aluminum pots and pans?" While possible connections between aluminum and Alzheimer's disease are still being studied, at this time there is no proven link between aluminum and dementia of the Alzheimer's type. If you have concerns about aluminum, you should ask a physician familiar with dementia to discuss them with you.

## Treatment of Alzheimer's Disease

There are at present no known ways to prevent or to cure Alzheimer's disease. This does not mean, however, that nothing can be done to relieve or reduce some of the symptoms of the disease, such as restlessness, anxiety, and difficulty sleeping. Medical management by a physician knowledgeable about Alzheimer's disease can assist in this regard. In addition, much can be done to provide stimulation, continued social interaction, healthful exercise, and enjoyable activity for your family member. Strategies can be learned that will reduce problem behaviors. Communication at the level of the affected person's changing capabilities can be encouraged and maintained. There is hope that your relative's life can continue to be meaningful and your life made easier despite the difficult challenges of Alzheimer's disease.

## References

Aronson, M. K. (Ed.) Alzheimer's Disease and Related Disorders Association. (1988). *Alzheimer's disease: What it is; how*

*to cope with it; future directions.* New York: Charles Scribner's Sons.

Cohen, D., & Eisdorfer, C. (1986). *The loss of self.* New York: W. W. Norton.

Mortimer, J. A., Schuman, L. M., & French, L. R. (1981). Epidemiology of dementing illness. In J. A. Mortimer & L. M. Schuman (Eds.), *The epidemiology of dementia.* New York: Oxford University Press.

Powell, L. S., & Courtice, K. (1983). *Alzheimer's disease: A guide for families.* Reading, MA: Addison-Wesley.

# Chapter 3

# Communication in Early Alzheimer's Disease

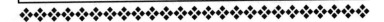

In the early stages of progressive dementia, communication changes may be subtle, and their onset gradual. Changes in recent memory, in the ability to pay attention and to concentrate, and in personality may combine to affect communication. Communication problems in this early phase are related to short-term memory loss, the length of the message, reduced attention and concentration, and an overall slowed ability to take in information. Some individuals will have significant problems with communication as the first (and for a time the only) sign of a dementing illness, but this is rare. This chapter describes some of the early changes in speaking and understanding seen in Alzheimer's disease, and Chapter 7 suggests some strategies for dealing with them.

# Changes in Communication: Early Signs

## Word-Finding Problems

One of the earliest indications of communication decline in Alzheimer's disease may be difficulty finding the right word, or remembering the name of a specific object. This is an early symptom common to most people with progressive dementia. These difficulties may be noticeable both in conversation and when the individual is responding to questions. At this stage, your family member may use his own strategies to help you understand what he is looking for. For example, he may say "I can't find that black thing I fix my hair with." Semantically "empty" words (such as "thing" and "stuff") may be used in place of specific words that are elusive. Communication may be lacking in information *content*.

Speech is generally still characterized by complete sentences and logical thoughts in these early stages. Long and unusual pauses between words may be noticeable, however, as the person requires more time to find words. It is important to keep in mind, though, that most of us have difficulty retrieving words at times. If this is the only communication difficulty you notice in your family member, it is not necessarily a sign of Alzheimer's disease!

## Comprehension Problems

In dementia's early stages, the ability to understand simple and concrete information is intact. In contrast, the ability to understand more abstract language, such as figures of speech, proverbs, and idioms is poor even in the beginning phases of the disease. Your family member may also have problems in following complex conversations and may appear to be "lost" in some communication exchanges. Other problems, such as hearing difficulty, can also result in comprehension difficulties, or make them worse for the person with dementia.

## Digression and Repeating

Because of difficulty with coming up with words and with following complex conversations, the person in the early stages of dementia will have a tendency to digress, or wander off track in conversations, at least for a short time. He will usually get back to the subject at hand without prompting, however. Problems with short-term memory will result in repetitions of stories or other infor-

mation perhaps only recently shared. This tendency of individuals with mild dementia to repeat themselves can be
very annoying and frustrating to family members. It calls
for the exercise of great patience — not an easy task!

## Writing and Reading

If the person with mild dementia has been a letter writer,
he will probably show early signs of difficulty with this
communication task and with other activities that require him to generate writing on his own. The mechanics of writing, however, will be intact. Although reading
comprehension problems may not be apparent, the person with mild dementia may show a diminished interest
in reading. This will be especially obvious if the individual was previously an avid or regular reader.

## Talking on the Telephone

Communicating over the telephone is a complicated activity. It requires that the person understand the message
coming over the phone; organize his thoughts to write
down the message if it needs to be remembered or given
to someone else; find the tools necessary to take down the
message (paper and pen or pencil); write down the message accurately, with its essential details; and remember
to pass on the message if necessary. If he is the one making the call, it also requires the ability to remember or to
look up the needed telephone number.

Communication over the telephone, especially the accurate relaying of messages and looking up phone num-

bers, can be very difficult for the person with even early, or mild, Alzheimer's disease. As the disease and its effects worsen, the person may not be able to use the telephone at all. It's important to keep in mind that your family member may not be able to successfully manage telephone messages, even though he still does quite well in face-to-face conversations.

## Awareness of Communication Difficulty

The person with mild dementia can be acutely aware of his verbal communication difficulties. He may joke about them to "cover up," or offer excuses when they occur. Especially in this early phase, your family member may express feelings of anger and frustration at what is happening to his mental functions and communication. The person's need to express these feelings and to talk about what is happening to him can be very strong. On the other hand, denial that anything is amiss may be the person's way of coping with the diagnosis and with feelings of confusion and loss of control that early cognitive changes bring.

## A Reminder About the Progression of Dementia

It is important to keep in mind, for your sake and the sake of your family member, that great individual differences exist in the *rate* at which dementia and the loss of communication skills progress, although the overall *pattern* of communication decline tends to be similar. Your relative may remain at the level of relatively mild dementia for months to years. If the disease is progressing slowly, the person with a diagnosis of dementia may remain quite a competent communicator for an extended period of time. At the same time, while people with Alzheimer's disease tend to show a similar *pattern* of decline of language functions, individual differences are seen. It will be important to take note of your family member's communication *strengths* as well as his deficiencies and to make use of those strengths to sustain communication.

## Formal Evaluations Can Be Helpful

If you live in a community where a variety of health care specialists are available, you may want to consider periodic evaluations by a *speech-language pathologist* familiar with dementia (perhaps every 6 months, or yearly). This individual can help to identify communication abilities that are still working well and those that are declining. Such information may assist you and other family members to develop effective strategies for communicating with the individual with dementia. If such services are not readily available, at least an initial assessment of communication abilities following the diagnosis of dementia can be helpful.

Regular assessments of memory and other cognitive abilities (again every 6 months or yearly) by a *neuropsychologist* will provide important information about changes in memory, thinking abilities, and judgment. This information can help you and your family member develop compensations for declining abilities and appreciate those skills that are still relatively intact. It's often easier to see the negative than the positive when dealing with progressive illness.

Health care professionals with knowledge of dementia can assist you in keeping your perspective, given the great variation among people in the rate of decline and pattern of abilities affected in dementia. If such services are not available in your community, or if you aren't sure how to go about locating them, you might ask your family member's physician for assistance or consult some of the resources listed in Chapter 17.

# Chapter 4

# Communication in the Middle Stages of Alzheimer's Disease

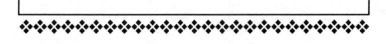

As dementing illness progresses, loss of memory and thinking abilities becomes more obvious. There is a marked reduction in the person's fund of factual knowledge, though old memories will still be relatively intact. The affected individual will begin to show an obvious decline in his ability to complete daily tasks, such as reading a book, following a recipe, doing household chores, using a telephone book, or shopping for groceries. He may be having difficulty keeping himself clean. His checkbook, if he is still keeping it, will most likely be in a sorry state. Your family member may now become lost in unfamiliar places and be unable to travel alone, though he will still recognize familiar surroundings.

You may notice with concern that your relative has begun to withdraw from previously enjoyed social activities, such as card games or get-togethers with friends. Problem behaviors may become more frequent. These can include being anxious and fearful, easily upset, uncharacteristically angry, and/or restless. (See Chapter 15 for more about how problem behaviors and communication difficulties may be related.)

In the middle stages of dementia, communication problems overall will be more frequent and more severe. Difficulties with understanding messages or expressing thoughts will increase in stressful, unfamiliar, or confusing situations. Repetitious questions and statements will be more frequent (and more annoying). Despite these problems, your relative may still continue to communicate quite effectively in familiar, comfortable surroundings and with familiar people until late in this middle stage. Specific changes in communication abilities that you may notice include the following: increasing difficulty finding words, declining verbal understanding, more obvious difficulty keeping conversations going, and withdrawal from speaking situations. Each of these communication changes is discussed in some detail in the following sections. At the same time, many of the social aspects of language use will remain intact, such as the ability to exchange greetings, to thank someone when appropriate, and to use the everyday pleasantries of conversation.

# Vocabulary and Word-Finding Abilities

Difficulty in finding specific words will be more frequent and more obvious as dementia progresses. You may notice that your relative often substitutes a closely related or associated word for the word he intends. For example, he may ask you to pass the sugar when he means the salt, or ask for a book when he wants a piece of paper. He may not necessarily show awareness of these verbal mistakes at this stage. These word substitutions are called *paraphasias.* Your relative will not be as efficient any more at "talking around" the word or name he cannot retrieve. You will find yourself guessing more, or playing "Twenty Questions" as you try to decipher what it is he would like to drink.

## Verbal Comprehension

Signs of worsening comprehension of verbal messages are characteristic of middle-stage dementia. Your relative may ask you to repeat your sentence several times before he indicates by his response that he has understood. The individual with moderate dementia will have obvious trouble following directions. He may need to have complex instructions broken into individual steps or require verbal "coaching" to complete such tasks as getting dressed or taking a bath.

## Maintaining Conversations

It will be more obvious in the middle stages of Alzheimer's disease that the affected person is losing the ability to participate in meaningful conversations. He may abruptly digress from the topic of discussion and not return to it unless prompted. He will have difficulty reestablishing his train of thought, and will leave sentences unfinished. Toward the end of the middle stage, your relative may appear to just "free associate." Increasingly frequently, he may seem to be speaking nonsense or "gibberish."

## Withdrawal from Speaking Situations

As Alzheimer's disease progresses, your family member will gradually begin to withdraw from conversational opportunities. He may stop initiating conversations and become less talkative. He may no longer be able to pick up on the conversation starters people typically employ, such as, "It sure is a lovely day today." He may not always respond when others speak to him. At this point, his sense of what is appropriate to keep a conversation going has begun to erode. He may appear uninterested or depressed when, in fact, he may no longer be able to participate in conversations.

## Social Aspects of Language

People with moderate dementia still appreciate the social uses of language. They maintain the ability to use cliches and expressions of social exchange appropriately. You may notice that your family member is still quite capable of shifting the topic of conversation away from himself when he hasn't understood a question asked of him. For example, he may say "I feel just fine! And how are you?" when asked by a nurse if he is in pain. People who only see you and your family member occasionally may have an overly optimistic impression of his communication abilities. He looks and sounds good in these brief social encounters.

Maintaining communication with your loved one as he moves through the moderate or middle stages of his illness becomes increasingly challenging. Chapter 8 offers you some strategies for sustaining interaction in the face of significant losses of memory and communication abilities.

# $C$hapter 5

# Communication in Severe Alzheimer's Disease

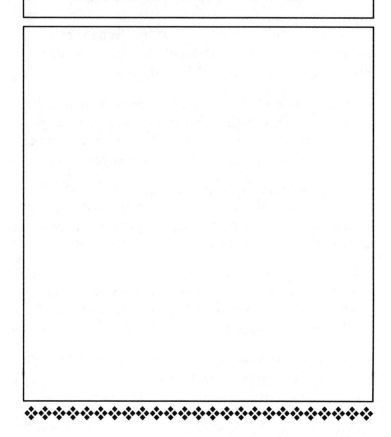

As the person with dementia moves into the more severe phases of the disease, he will begin to require physical assistance with the basic activities of daily living, such as dressing, bathing, eating, and grooming. He will begin to have noticeable motor problems and may need to have some assistance with walking. Chewing and swallowing food become difficult for most dementia victims at some point in the disease, in part because they "forget" that they need to swallow. In the final stages of dementing illness, the person will require assistance with all basic daily life activities. Emotional expression will be minimal, and bladder and bowel incontinence (lack of control) is common. The person may retain only the remnants of knowledge about his past life. Communication difficulties are profound in these final stages of the disease. They are summarized below:

1. In the moderate-to-severe phase of Alzheimer's disease, the person with dementia expresses his thoughts and feelings in more and more basic terms. Sentence structures become simplified and less complete.

2. The person may be extremely limited in his ability to make even basic needs known. In the last stages of dementia, he may be no longer capable of communicating these needs at all.

3. As memory for the meaning of even common words further erodes, verbal comprehension problems are severe. In the late stages of the disease, verbal understanding is minimal.

4. Expressive vocabulary is severely reduced and increasingly "empty," or imprecise.

5. If the person is still able to speak, he may babble, utter the same sound or word repetitively, or echo another speaker. Responses, if present, will consist of repetitious phrases and one-word responses.

6. Some basic pragmatics, or social aspects of language, may be spared in people with severe dementia. For example, they may respond on an automatic or reflexive level with "Thank you" and "Please," or say "How nice!" when you bring them a treat.

Even in the severe and final stages of Alzheimer's disease, when the afflicted person's abilities to speak and understand are minimal, there are things you can do to communicate your care and affection in nonverbal ways. Chapter 9 offers some suggestions that may be useful.

# Chapter 6

## Keeping Communication Channels Open: General Principles and Guidelines

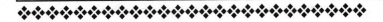

This chapter discusses some ideas for maintaining and improving communication with your family member at any stage in the progression of Alzheimer's disease or a related dementia. They are general principles of "good communication" that can be applied in most situations. These general guidelines are a good place to start if communicating with your loved one is becoming difficult or if you want to build your communication skills in preparation for probable difficult times ahead.

In most interactions, both (or all) of the people involved take some responsibility for maintaining communication. For example, we clarify what we mean, express our point of view, ask questions, or provide information. The situation is much different, however, when one of the parties has a disease that progressively affects memory, new learning, communication abilities, personality, and judgment. As the caregiver of a person with Alzheimer's disease, the responsibility for maintaining and nurturing communication as long as possible rests with you. Observing these rules of good communication should make that task easier, at least most of the time. It will also allow your loved one to use his communication skills to the best of his ability, for as long as possible.

# How to Maintain Communication

Creating a positive communication environment is the first step in helping your family member maintain his dignity and self-worth and in making your caregiving tasks easier. Following are some general suggestions for maintaining communication.

## Eliminate Background Noise

Alzheimer's disease and other dementias affect a person's ability to pay attention, to concentrate, and to "screen out" unwanted background noise and other distractions. When you want to communicate with your family member, turn down or turn off the television and the radio. Choose a quiet room or environment for your conversation, if possible, but especially for important communications. Your relative will be able to attend to your message and to hear you better if these distractions are reduced.

## Be Sure You Have the Person's Attention

Get your family member's attention *before* you begin to speak. Some ways to do this are to say his name, or get his attention with a gentle touch on the arm. Don't try to communicate information when the person with dementia is concentrating on completing another task or when unavoidable distractions are competing for his attention. *Especially important is not to simply call out to him from another room!* The confused person may become even more disoriented and confused if he cannot identify the source of the voice he hears.

## Establish and Maintain Good Eye Contact

Look directly at your relative and position yourself on his eye level, when possible. In this way, you're allowing the person with dementia to benefit from the visual cues of your facial expression and mouth movements, and you have the added information of his facial expressions and speech movements. These visual cues are important in communication.

## Be a Patient Listener

People even in the beginning stages of a progressive dementia often need more time to retrieve the word they're looking for, or to express a particular thought. Rather than supplying the word, if what the person needs is a little more time, give him that time. This is not always easy to do, especially if you are feeling rushed in the middle of a busy day. But keep in mind that no one likes to be interrupted when speaking, or to have someone else put words in his mouth!

## Be Generous With Your Approval

As the caregiver of someone with dementia, it's important to keep in mind that it is *you,* and not your family member who sets the standard for what is a "good enough" performance. You establish "the height of the bar" over which he has to climb, so to speak. This applies just as much to his communication attempts or to how well he remembers what you've recently told him as it does to how neatly he shaves himself. You must decide whether it really matters that he put on two shirts today instead of just one, given the fact that he did dress himself. Your family member may be trying hard for your approval as he struggles to accomplish even simple tasks. Be generous!

## Be an Active and Creative Listener

Even in the early stages of dementing illness there may be times when your relative is having difficulty expressing himself clearly. You will need to listen to the "gist" of the message, because the actual words that are coming out may be confusing. Learn to focus on the thought or feeling that your family member is trying to express. His facial expression, tone of voice, and body language may help you interpret the message.

## Maintain the Person's Dignity

Remember that the person with Alzheimer's disease is still an adult with feelings and perceptions despite loss of memory and other abilities. Avoid "talking down" to the person as you would to a child, even though you may need to simplify messages. Above all, do not talk about your family member to others in his presence, as if he were not there or did not understand. It is difficult to tell just how much a person with dementia understands, especially in the later stages of the illness. It is best to assume that he is understanding and to incorporate him into the conversation as much as possible. For example, it is better to say "John, your friend Frank Johnson has stopped by to see us" than to say "Frank, John doesn't remember who you are. His memory is really getting bad."

## Be a Sensitive Listener

Don't call attention to the verbal mistakes your relative makes by challenging them or correcting them. If he attempts to hide his verbal slips, permit him this face-saving gesture. Don't mock or laugh at these verbal slips. If you've understood the message, you can let the wrong word go by.

## Use a Calm Tone of Voice

Maintaining a calm, relaxed attitude in communication exchanges is important and will be reflected in your voice. A high-pitched voice communicates stress, whereas a calm voice and slightly lower pitch help you sound more relaxed. Your calm, relaxed speaking style will assist your relative to maintain the focus on your conversation without anxiety that you may be angry or upset with him. Listen to how *you* sound in conversations with your family member. Your emotions as reflected in your voice (angry? frustrated? calm and in control?) will influence how the person with dementia responds to your communication.

## Watch Your Body Language

Body language is a powerful aspect of communication. Tense neck muscles, clenched fists, and a worried, tense facial expression will communicate frustration, anger, or worry to your relative, despite your calm words. Be aware of what your "body language" is communicating to the impaired person. Work to develop some relaxation techniques and strategies that you can apply when you're feeling stressed.

## Become a Good Observer

It will be very important that, as time goes on, you learn to become a careful observer in communication exchanges with your relative. You will need to identify signs and symptoms of communication difficulty, or what circumstances trigger breakdowns in communication. Is your relative showing signs of fatigue and overstimulation when communication falters? Is communication more difficult after a tiring day, or when you have a house full of company? Did your family member not seem to understand what you were asking him to do? What adjustments on your part seem to improve communication (for example, speaking more slowly, giving one-step requests or directions, using simple, direct statements)? Does your relative give indications that he is aware of his communication difficulties? As you become more observant about what factors help or hinder communication with your family member, you'll be better able to plan ahead to anticipate potential difficulties and apply successful coping strategies.

## Take Care of Any Sensory Problems

Individuals with Alzheimer's disease are not immune to the decreases in hearing and vision that may affect all of us as we age. Sensory deficits, such as poor hearing or limited vision, can make someone with dementia appear as if he is more cognitively impaired than is actually the case. Treating these problems will help the person with dementia to function within his true remaining cognitive abilities.

If you suspect that your family member may have an untreated hearing loss, or that hearing functions have gotten worse, help him arrange for an appropriate medical evaluation. Make an appointment with a physician who specializes in the medical treatment of diseases of the ear (an ENT physician, or *otolaryngologist*). You will also want to have his hearing evaluated by a professional who measures and diagnoses hearing disorders (an *audiologist*). The audiologist also provides nonmedical treatment for the communication problems associated with hearing loss (for example, counseling regarding hearing aid use).

If your family member has never worn a hearing aid, and you think that a hearing aid might help, it is important to pursue a hearing evaluation as early as possible after a diagnosis of probable Alzheimer's disease has been made. As the dementia progresses, it becomes more difficult for the person to adjust to changes and to cope with new learning, such as would be necessary for successful adjustment to a hearing aid. Chances of success are better if a hearing aid is introduced in the early stages of the disease. For more information on coping with hearing loss, you may want to refer to another volume in this series, *Coping with Hearing Loss and Hearing Aids,* by Debra A. Shimon.

If you are concerned that visual problems are preventing your family member from functioning at his best, you will want to make an appointment with a physician who specializes in diagnosing and treating diseases of the eye (an *ophthalmologist*). If medical or surgical treatment (such as cataract surgery) is not recommended, an evaluation of the person's current eyeglass prescription needs may be made by a nonmedical professional (an *optometrist*).

Finally, if your relative has a hearing aid and/or eyeglasses, make sure they are in good working order and readily available. Learn how to troubleshoot the hearing aid, and have replacement batteries on hand. If others are sharing the care of your loved one, let them know how important these sensory aids are to him. In the face of a progressive dementia, it is easy to overlook those devices that will assist your family member to function better as a communicator.

# Chapter 7

# Communication Strategies in the Early Stages of Dementia

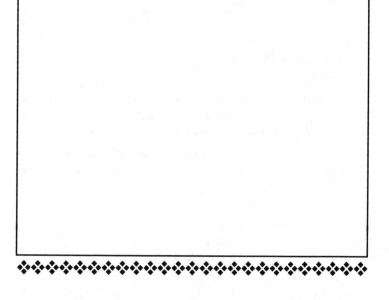

This chapter offers some specific suggestions to assist your family member in his communicative efforts and to help you structure your own ways of communicating with him in the early phases of dementia. Some suggestions are designed to assist your relative's failing memory abilities, while others more directly relate to verbal interactions. Remember that it won't necessarily be easy for you to change your lifelong habits of talking and listening, so don't be too hard on yourself if you're not always the model of patient listening and clear, simple speaking. On the other hand, these are behaviors that *can* be learned. Once these communication strategies are learned and put into practice, understanding the person with mild dementia and assisting him to understand you will become easier.

## Suggestions for Dealing with Memory Difficulties

Problems with short-term memory (memory for recent events and recently presented information) are closely related to some of the communication difficulties seen early in dementing illness. In fact, failing short-term memory helps to explain many of the communication problems observed in the early stages of dementia. The following ideas include techniques and strategies that aid memory and that should also serve to improve communication.

## Repeat Messages Frequently

Because the person with dementia demonstrates difficulty remembering information over a span of minutes to hours, you will need to repeat your messages frequently. This can be done unobtrusively and without "blaming" the person for his failing memory. For example, you might say in the morning, "Bob and Mary Thompson have invited us to go on a picnic with them this afternoon." A short while later, you may say, "I'm making a salad to take on the picnic this afternoon. The Thompsons are picking us up." Still later, you might say, "Perhaps it would be a good idea to rest a little before we go to the picnic this afternoon. Wasn't it nice of Bob and Mary Thompson to invite us."

## Use Memory Aids

Encourage the person with mild dementia to use written reminders of appointments, upcoming events, or items to be purchased. A calendar or a daily schedule posted in an easily seen place in the home can be helpful. If your family member has shown an inclination for keeping a daily diary or journal, encourage him to continue to do this as long as possible. It can be a helpful memory tool and reference source as things are forgotten.

## Provide Information Close to the Time Needed

Don't give specific directions, instructions, or other important information too far in the future. Provide this information to your family member as close as possible to the time when it is actually needed. Otherwise, you'll be tiring yourself out and find that you have to repeat information more often than is necessary. You might say, "It's time to put your coat on now. We're ready to leave for your doctor's appointment" instead of reminding your family member about his coat 45 minutes before you need to leave. Of course, you've prepared him for the trip to the doctor by reminders about that throughout the day.

# Suggestions to Assist Verbal Comprehension

As the brain's ability to process information begins to slow, and attention and concentration become more difficult, the person with early-stage dementia can benefit from the strategies you adopt to structure your communication with him. Below are some suggestions for enhancing comprehension that might work in your situation. Review the general suggestions offered in Chapter 6 as well.

## Structure Conversations

You can assist the person with early-stage dementia to better follow conversations by beginning them in a casual, friendly manner and by structuring the information you present. Remember to use information that will help orient him to the topic right at the beginning. The conversation might be about a current local or state election issue, or neighborhood concern, for example. First, *introduce the topic.* You might begin by saying, "This is a request for the city to put a stoplight at the corner of our street and Walnut Avenue." Second, *provide an overview of the topic or issue.* "Our neighbors, the Browns, brought it by for us to sign. People in the neighborhood are upset at all of the traffic accidents that have been happening on that corner." Finally, *fill in the details.* "There's going to be a neighborhood meeting about it this Thursday evening at 7:30. Would you like to go?" The principle involved in structuring the conversation is to go from the general to the specific. Keep in mind that even the person with mild memory and processing difficulties will have trouble "putting the pieces together" in following a conversation.

## Use Simple, Direct Language

Statements that are worded in the *active voice* (for example, "Bob drives the car") are easier to understand and to process than statements that utilize the *passive voice* (for example, "The car is driven by Bob"). Likewise, literal language is easier for the person with memory and other cognitive deficits to process than are idioms, metaphors, and other figures of speech. Your family member will understand verbal messages more easily if you use direct language, short simple sentences, and the active voice. Express more complex thoughts in several shorter, simple sentences. In time, you will also have to simplify the vocabulary you use. The challenge is to speak simply and directly, without patronizing or "talking down" to the communicatively impaired person.

## Learn the Limits of the Person's Attention and Concentration Span

Even in these early stages, it's important to observe and learn the limits of your relative's attention span for conversation or other language activities. You'll develop a sense of when to suggest a rest period, or some quiet time, and when to end a particular conversation. Let your family member's behavior guide you on this.

# Suggestions for Encouraging Verbal Expression

The individual who is experiencing the early stages of dementia may be aware that he is having trouble finding the right word or expressing his thoughts clearly. This can be a source of frustration, anger, and concern. At times when communication is difficult, the following strategies may be helpful.

### Encourage Circumlocution

When we describe a person whose name we cannot recall at the moment, or relate the plot and the stars of a movie whose title temporarily eludes us, we are using *circumlocution,* that is, "talking around" the word or words that are unavailable. This can be an effective technique for the person with mild dementia. Encourage your family member to describe the particular item he wants, or for which he's searching. Ask if he can tell you in a "different way," or with other words. Ask if he can tell you "something else" about the item, place, or person. With this additional information, you can often interpret the person's attempts to communicate. When this strategy is successful, point this out to your loved one. Reinforce or compliment the use of this technique. Suggest ways that this strategy can be used in daily conversations.

## Allow Time for Processing

The individual in the early stages of dementing illness may frequently be able to come up with the desired word, or express what is on his mind if given a little more time. For the person with mild dementia, this extra time to express himself may be all that is needed in many communicative situations.

## Keep the Conversation on Track

During conversations, the person with dementia may seem to "drift" from the topic at hand and not always come back to it. To get the conversation back on track, remind him tactfully of the topic you had been discussing. When there is an opportunity to break into the conversation unobtrusively, summarize or rephrase in your own words what you understood the person to be saying before he got sidetracked.

## Let Him Reminisce

At the same time, it is beneficial to let your family member digress a bit, and to reminisce. This keeps him verbally communicating with you and a part of the conversation. You can gently bring him back to the topic when necessary. Recalling past times and events in his life may be one of his best communication skills now.

## Provide Opportunities to Express Feelings

Allow your family member opportunities to talk about his feelings with regard to his disease: loss of previously taken-for-granted abilities, anger that this is happening to him, frustration when memory fails or communication becomes difficult, and fear of abandonment in the future. The person with mild dementia will likely share his feelings if given the opportunity. Attentive listening strategies are especially important here. Be tuned in to when your relative *wants* to talk about what he is feeling or when he expresses concerns and anxieties about his condition. Your goal is to understand the feelings behind the statements.

The challenge will be to respond with positive and reassuring comments when your relative expresses concerns. Respond with empathy and a warm, supportive tone of voice to his expressed feelings. At the same time, your responses must be realistic and not stifle conversations dealing with concerns and feelings. Don't argue with your family member if he says such things as, "I know there's no cure for this," or "Nothing can be done to help me." Avoid getting into a contest of wills where the person taking one side of an argument has to lose.

Instead, find something positive and reassuring to say about the fact that the individual is supported and loved, that he shows courage and determination, and that each day can be lived as fully as possible. If you are asked whether things "will get worse," acknowledge gently that this is the case, but that the person still has many strengths. Remind your family member about some recently enjoyed activity or pleasant event. Stress that together you'll share each day as it comes.

## Should I Tell Him He Has Alzheimer's Disease?

The issue of whether to share with your family member his diagnosis of Alzheimer's disease is a troublesome one for many caregivers. One question to ask yourself is, has he asked? If he has raised the question specifically, you can and should answer in a straightforward manner. For example, "Yes, that is what your doctor has told us." How much more detail to share should be guided by the questions your family member asks. There is no need to tell him everything you've read about the end stages of the illness because he has asked whether what is happening to him has a name. You may find that your loved one accepts the answer to his question matter-of-factly. He is likely to be satisfied with a brief explanation.

There is another good reason for considering telling your relative that he has Alzheimer's disease. If family energies are being directed to keeping the diagnosis a secret from the person most directly affected, this can influence social interactions and postpone planning for the future. No one around the person with dementia wants to slip and say the words "Alzheimer's disease," but those words are in the background just the same.

If you are having trouble dealing with the issue of what to tell your relative about his disease, talk with his physician, or with the dementia team if one is available to you. They can help. If you are participating in a dementia caregiver support group, bring up the question there. It may help you to see how others have handled the delicate question of what and how much to share with the person with dementia.

## Consider Group Involvement

You may want to explore whether there are groups available in your community for people with recently diagnosed, mild Alzheimer's disease. Having the chance to come together with other memory-disordered individuals may have a therapeutic effect in helping your family member learn strategies for managing current problems and difficulties. A support group setting offers an opportunity to share in an understanding and accepting environment.

Some health care professionals recommend including mildly memory-impaired people in mixed groups, with others whose memories are still intact but who might have other difficulties or concerns. Such groups can provide appropriate stimulation and activity for the person with mild dementia. Inquire as to what types of groups might be available in your community.

## Provide Stimulating Language Activities

Language-based activities such as word games (Scrabble, Hangman, Twenty Questions, Trivia), crossword puzzles, and similar activities provide excellent vocabulary and word-retrieval stimulation. If your family member enjoyed these types of activities prior to his illness, encourage their continued use. Books of jokes and limericks can still be enjoyed at this stage of progressive dementia.

## Use Questions to Stimulate Conversation and Involvement

Using questions involving choice to stimulate conversation will help keep your family member communicatively engaged. If you have taken your relative shopping with you, for example, you might ask, "Do you think the flowered towels or the striped towels are prettier?" or "Do you like the dark blue, or the maroon shirt?" The goal in asking such questions is to *include* the person in the conversation, and to stimulate memory and thinking, not to "test" him. *Never let the conversation turn into a "drill" activity by putting your family member on the spot with frequent questions!*

# When the Person with Dementia Lives Alone

When the person with mild dementia is still living on his own, some special issues regarding communication need to be addressed. For example, you may have concerns about whether he can still manage telephone communication and whether he can understand and deal with written material such as bills, instructions for taking medicines, and advertisements. You may, on the other hand, already be assisting your family member with paying bills and managing his checkbook.

## Communicating on the Telephone

You will want to be sure that your family member can still communicate adequately by telephone when he needs assistance. Look for an opportunity to check and see if he is able to look up numbers in his personal telephone directory and dial the necessary sequence of numbers. If he is unsure or inconsistent in being able to do these things, there are telephones available now that let you program several important numbers into the phone's memory. All the impaired person needs to do is press one button and the number is dialed for him. Each button can be labeled to identify whose number it dials. Some phones come with large, easy-to-read numbers.

You may also want to check to see whether your relative is still able to use a telephone book. If he can't, you might think of ways to simplify the task. For example, make a list of numbers he is likely to need and program those into a telephone such as the one just described. Be sure to include important emergency numbers.

You should do some role-playing with your relative, if he is agreeable, to confirm that he can summon the appropriate person or agency when needed. Describe a situation such as, "If you needed me to come right over, how would you dial my number?" or "Which button dials my number?" Another role-playing example could be "Which button would you push to get help quickly if you were in trouble?" Have him show you that he can contact you and other family members, as well as specific emergency numbers.

Some communities also have emergency contact systems, such as Lifeline, that are available for a monthly charge. These systems allow someone to summon assistance even if they are physically unable to get to a phone. For the person with dementia, the important question is whether he can understand the purpose of such a system and how and when to use it. You can inquire about such services through your local aging services agency, hospital social work department, or similar organizations.

## Understanding Written Material

It is important for you to know whether your relative who lives alone can understand the reading material that comes into his home. You may have questions such as: Does he understand that this is a bill to be paid? Does he understand the fine print in this advertisement? Will he be able to follow the directions for taking his medicine, if I print them in large-size print?

If your family member is already letting you help with responding to mail, paying bills, going over written directions, and advising on purchases, the question may not be so crucial. If he is still handling these tasks himself, however, you need to get at least a general idea about his reading ability.

Some ways to approach this casually (and without seeming to put him on the spot) might be the following:

1. Go over some short articles or advertisements in the newspaper. Have your family member read a few sentences and tell you about what he has just read.

2. Ask him to tell you about particular pieces of mail, if he shares his mail with you.

3. Have him explain to you how often, how much, and when he is supposed to take a particular medicine. If he has trouble taking medicines accurately, a pharmacist can help you set up a simplified system for him.

## Other Resources

If you still have concerns about your relative's ability to manage some communication situations on his own, other help may be available. *Speech-language pathologists* can evaluate reading comprehension and the ability to use the telephone. *Occupational therapists* are health care professionals who do evaluations that indicate how well and how safely a person can manage a variety of tasks in the home. They also can provide advice on what types of aids and devices will allow someone to continue to be as independent as possible, as well as suggestions for making tasks easier to accomplish. County or private *home health agencies* can be good sources for finding out whether these services are available in your area.

# Chapter 8

# Communication Strategies in the Middle Stages of Dementia

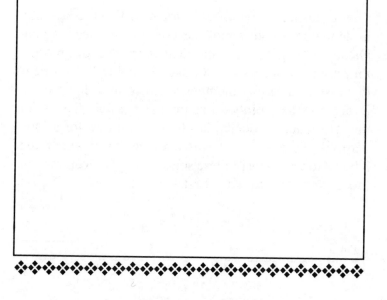

The suggestions found in this chapter will help assure that communication successes are maintained during the middle, or moderate, stages of Alzheimer's disease. Let's first review the description of the declines in communication abilities apparent at this stage. Your family member is becoming a more dependent communicator, as he requires you to "guess" and interpret the sometimes garbled messages he communicates. At the same time, he has become more dependent on you for other support as well: transportation, assistance with daily living needs, and direction and guidance to prevent wandering and getting lost in unfamiliar places. In addition, a large part of your energies must now go into making sure that your family member understands what is wanted of him and that he comprehends important messages. As your relative becomes a less effective communicator, you will need to become his advocate in many interactions with those professionals assisting you in his care. A large, sometimes seemingly overwhelming job!

The suggestions offered below are based on the fact that, as dementia becomes more severe, you will need to plan ahead and structure communicative interactions more if they are to be successful. An overall goal in this phase is to assist your family member to function at his present levels of verbal ability for as long as possible. This middle, or moderate, dementia phase can go on for a long while. With practice, it will become easier and more natural to use some of these suggestions. Concentrate on those that seem to work best for you.

# Coping with Increasingly Severe Memory Problems

Memory deficits will become more obvious and more severe in the middle stages of Alzheimer's disease. You will want to organize the environment to compensate for your family member's failing ability to remember information. The following ways of structuring the environment can ease communication by assisting the person to remember familiar daily routines and specific information.

## Develop a Predictable Daily Routine

One of the most universal pieces of advice given to care providers of memory-impaired adults is to establish a predictable daily routine. As much as possible, plan for meals, naps, walks or other exercise to occur at the same time every day. Plan for such tasks as baths at a regular time as well. It will be of great help in setting up a daily schedule to observe when your relative seems most open to social interaction, to exercising, or to resting. An ideal daily schedule will take into account the impaired person's past preferences and "daily rhythms." It will not only help your relative to have a predictable daily schedule; it can greatly ease your job as well. Eliminating confusion and unpredictability in day-to-day activities will help reduce your family member's anxiety and increase his cooperation. It will help to create an environment in which communication can still occur.

Of course it won't be possible to structure every day in the same way, never veering from the daily schedule. When something out of the ordinary is to occur, prepare the person with dementia by providing specific reminders ("Today, the children are coming over." "This morning, I need to go grocery shopping. Bill is coming over to keep you company."). If you notice, however, that the anticipation of an upcoming event begins to preoccupy your relative, avoid these reminders.

## Label the Environment

As time passes, it will become increasingly difficult for the person with dementia to remember where familiar items are kept. Some caregivers find it helpful to label drawers, closets, and other storage places with their contents as a help to their relative in finding and replacing items. This strategy will only work, of course, if the affected person is still able to read *and understand* written words. You might, for example, label bedroom drawers with "socks," "underwear," "sweaters," and so forth. Kitchen drawers and cupboards labeled with their contents might allow your family member to continue to help with such tasks as setting the table and putting away the dishes. Labeling the home environment may not work for everyone, but if providing such cues to the affected person reduces repetitive questions and allows the individual to function more independently and securely, it's worth a try.

# Assisting Verbal Comprehension

In the middle stages of dementia, semantic memory, or the memory for the meaning of words and ideas, is further disrupted. Because of this loss of semantic memory, your relative will have more difficulty understanding spoken messages. You'll be more successful in getting through to him if you incorporate some of the following suggestions into your conversations.

## Adjust Your Vocabulary

As communication with your relative becomes more challenging, you'll need to adapt the words you choose to his current ability to understand. Use concrete, specific, and simple words. Work at not introducing new vocabulary or unusual phrases in your communication with him. Instead of using words such as "this," "these," "he," and "she," use the name of the item or the specific person. Say, for example, "You need to put your shoes on now" rather than "Here, put these on" as you hand him the shoes. Refer to "your brother Tom" or "your cousin Betty" rather than to "he" or "she."

## Break Down Instructions into Steps

In the middle or moderate stages of dementia, the ability to follow through on routine tasks such as preparing a meal, setting the table, or hoeing the garden is impaired.

Your family member may need to be taken through the steps of even such basic activities of daily living as grooming himself and dressing. At this stage, it is important to *give one step or instruction at a time* if the person needs verbal cuing to complete an activity.

If there is an activity that your relative can no longer accomplish, think about the individual steps involved in completing the task. By breaking down the task into separate small steps and providing verbal cuing, he may be able to successfully complete the activity. A task that was confusing in its complexity to the person with moderate dementia may become manageable, less frustrating for both of you, and a measure of successful accomplishment when taken step by step. Remember how important it is to your relative's mobility, his overall fitness, and his self-esteem for him to care for himself and to remain independent. *People with dementia quickly become quite helpless if you do tasks for them.*

An example of how you might break down a task into its individual steps is the daily activity of assisting your family member to get dressed in the morning. It no longer works to simply say "It's time to get dressed." First, you may have to "coach" him to take off his pajamas before dressing. Next, you will need to verbally guide your relative to put on one item of clothing at a time. You may need to hand each item to him as you tell him what it is ("Here is your undershirt; here are your shorts").

Even though he now requires more help with the task of dressing, you can still give your relative some choices about what he wants to wear ("Would you like to wear your blue shirt, or the tan one?"). Another way to allow him some choice is to let him select a pair of pants from the closet or wardrobe, but have only two or three pair hanging there that day.

## Use Many Ways to Get your Message Across

As words lose their meaning and verbal messages become increasingly confusing to the person with dementia, you will need to make use of as many communication channels as possible to get your meaning across. Communicating will provide an opportunity to use your best thespian talents! Accompany your spoken instructions with friendly gestures, pictures, pantomiming with objects, and/or facial expression. Match your verbal message with the appropriate tone of voice and facial expression. Don't forget the communicative power of body language!

And don't forget to look for ways to *bring some humor* into your daily struggles to communicate. If the atmosphere can be lightened with a shared laugh, you both will benefit. Take advantage of opportunities to laugh at yourself or at a particular situation, not at the person with dementia.

In the later stages of moderate dementia, you may need to guide your family member with your hands in getting an activity started, such as combing his hair or feeding himself. Remember that communication doesn't mean just speaking, but also involves visual cues, gestures, and other ways of getting our meaning across.

## Provide Help with Shifts in Conversational Topics

For the individual with moderate dementia, following abrupt shifts in the topic of conversation will be difficult. In one-to-one conversations with your family member, you can provide "lead in" cues, such as, "Let's talk about _____ now." If it's a group conversation and your relative appears confused when the conversation has shifted, give him a brief explanation, for example, "Bob is telling us about his fishing trip last weekend." This can be done with subtlety and without embarrassment to the person with dementia.

# Encouraging Verbal Expression

As dementing illness progresses, your family member will find it more difficult to express his thoughts, feelings, and needs. Although you cannot replace lost communication skills, there are a number of things you *can* do to help his verbal expression. Here are some suggestions.

## Structure Your Questions

It is better to ask either/or questions than to ask open-ended ones when you want a response. For example, asking "Do you want coffee or a soda to drink, John?" is more likely to elicit an appropriate response than "What do you want to drink, John?" Avoid asking open-ended questions such as "Who called?" "What would you like to do?" "What do you need?" Instead, frame your questions in the following ways: "Was that Michael on the phone?" "Would you like to go for a walk now?" "Do you need some sugar and milk for your cereal?"

## Use Clues Available in the Situation

You can facilitate successful communication with the person with moderate dementia if you use your observational skills and let the context of the situation provide clues. When your relative is rummaging in his dresser drawer and it is cool in the house, asking "Are you looking for your sweater?" can elicit a smile of affirmation, whereas asking "What are you looking for?" may result in a puzzled look of confusion.

You will also pick up important clues as to your relative's intended message by listening *actively,* that is, paying attention to his facial expression, gestures, and tone of voice as well as to the words he is expressing. Can you pick up the *emotion* being expressed, even if the words aren't making total sense? Using *all* of the available contextual cues can result in a successful communicative interaction.

## Play "Twenty Questions"

Using a "Twenty Questions" format, which allows your family member to respond with "yes" or "no" can be helpful when you're trying to determine what he is trying to express. Be sure to ask just one question at a time, though! For example, you can ask, "Do you want something to drink?" if he is searching through the refrigerator or cupboard. If that elicits a positive response, you can go down the list of likely beverages, one at a time.

## Use Clues that the Person with Dementia can Provide

If your relative is still able to describe the item or person he is thinking of, or if he can tell you the category (for example, "I'm hungry. I want something to eat") ask him to describe the wanted item or tell you something else about the person of whom he's thinking. ("Do you want something hot, or something cold to eat?" "Is it a neighbor, or someone in the family you're thinking of?"). Ask him to use gestures to help you understand if he is able to do this ("Can you *show* me with your hands?"). These efforts will not only result in more successful communication efforts; they will also show your family member that you're trying to understand and to communicate with him. He'll be encouraged to keep interacting verbally.

## Ask Relevant Conversational Questions

Whereas the individual with mild dementia will, if given extra time, usually be able to bring himself back to the topic of conversation, the person in the moderate stages of dementia will need more structured help to tell his story. He will not only drift away from the conversational topic, but may not be aware he has done so, and may not be able to bring himself back to the topic at hand. You can assist to keep the conversation on track by asking relevant questions, by gently reminding your relative of what he was talking about ("You were telling me about what you did at the Senior Center today" or "You were mentioning how much you liked to go fishing when you were a boy"), and by paraphrasing and summarizing what you have understood of the conversation up to that point ("I think you're telling me that you don't feel very well. Is your stomach upset? Can you show me where it hurts?").

# Maintaining Social Interactions

Socializing with other people and communication are difficult to separate. Social interaction *is* communication. Withdrawal from social situations and a decline in attempts to communicate can both be seen in the middle stages of dementing illness. As the dementia progresses, you will want to assist your family member to maintain his ability to interact socially with others for as long as possible. Keeping up social contacts will be a considerable challenge for both of you as his ability to remember and to enjoy conversations fades. Utilize some of the suggestions that follow to keep your loved one interacting socially.

## Plan for Success

You will want to encourage those types of social interactions in which your family member can be successful. This will depend on his current level of language and communication skills, as well as on his attention and concentration span. Small gatherings that involve a few close friends or relatives are likely to work best. If a close friend or family member offers to take your relative out for a drive or to a ball game, accept the offer. Invite another couple or an individual over for a short visit and some refreshments. You'll have a good sense of whom to invite — those people your family member knows well and likes, who will be patient with and tolerant of his communication limitations, and who respect his dignity. Accept some invitations that include small numbers of old friends and close family. Be sure to watch for signs of fatigue, anxiety, or restlessness in your family member, because they can be signals that it's probably time to end the visit.

## Avoid Difficult Social Situations

Social gatherings that require interacting with strangers, that include unfamiliar activities, or that involve large groups of people are likely to be confusing and upsetting to your relative as dementia worsens. Imagine not being able to remember whether someone is a friend or a stranger, or whether you're supposed to remember this person or introduce yourself to him. How frightening such a situation must be when the underpinnings of memory are no longer working! Noisy parties, large family reunions, or having all of the children and grandchildren over at the same time will probably be frustrating and fatiguing for both of you. Instead, plan quiet times with the people you and he want to see, a few at a time.

## Continue to Stimulate Communication

There are many things you can do to continue to stimulate communicative interactions in the middle stages of dementia. Choose activities that your relative enjoys and that are successful for him. You might want to consider some of the following ideas:

1. Looking through family albums and talking about the people and events portrayed can help to recall pleasant times and stimulate old memories.

2. Listening to favorite music and singing along with old songs can be both an enjoyable and successful activity.

3. Taking walks together and talking about what you're seeing, or having a daily routine of some easy, gentle exercises to music or a videotape provide both healthful and enjoyable shared activity (you'll benefit from the exercise too!).

4. Your family member might still enjoy playing simple card games, even though he can no longer concentrate on Bridge or Pinochle.

5. Having a family pet to help care for can be stimulating and rewarding for the memory-impaired person. Advice usually given, however, is not to choose a dog or cat as a new pet for someone with dementia, because of the work involved in caring for such a pet. A small pet such as a bird or fish would be a better choice.

Many of the resources mentioned in Chapter 17 contain other specific suggestions for communication-centered activities appropriate for the person with moderate dementia. You'll come up with some of your own ideas as well, based on your family member's current capabilities, past and present interests, and available opportunities. The important thing to remember is that you want to keep his *desire* to communicate alive as long as possible.

# Chapter 9

# Maintaining Communication when Dementia is Severe

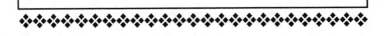

Communication with a person with severe dementia involves making use of whatever verbal or nonverbal channels remain to assure his comfort and safety, while at the same time maintaining affectionate contact and providing continued stimulation. When dementia has reached the severe to final stages, your family member will be totally dependent on you and others for his basic survival needs.

As was discussed in Chapter 5, in the severe stages of Alzheimer's disease speech will be only fragmentary, or absent altogether. Some repetitive single words or phrases may be heard. It is likely that the person fails to understand most things that are said to him, though some understanding of tone of voice, facial expression, and simple gestures (for example, holding out your hands for the person to grasp to help him get up) will remain.

It will become more difficult for you to know whether your loved one is comfortable or in pain, or whether he wants something to eat or drink. You'll become more skilled at picking up on small cues that your family member is uncomfortable or is satisfied. You'll need to be alert for signs of physical illness: infections, skin breakdown, or other medical problems that might warrant a call to his physician or nurse practitioner.

What can make these last phases of caring so difficult and stressful for you is that the person with severe dementia will likely require considerable physical care, yet at the same time he will be unable to understand the need for such care, to respond to you the caregiver, or to cooperate in caregiving tasks.

# Suggestions for Maintaining Communication

Some specific ideas for maintaining communicative contact with your loved one in the severe to final phases of his illness are offered below. Other suggestions can be found in the resources listed in Chapter 17.

## Maintain Social Exchange

Your relative can still comprehend on some level the everyday social exchanges people use with one another. Remember to greet him by name and to identify yourself every time you approach. As you leave his presence, remember to say and to wave goodbye. Ask him how he is feeling, or tell him that you hope he is feeling well, even though he may not be able to respond with words. You will help maintain his dignity as a person by remembering these small but important gestures of social communication.

## Keep Talking

As a person becomes a less able communication partner, we have a natural tendency to talk less to him, to have fewer verbal interactions. It's uncomfortable to keep talking to someone who cannot respond to us verbally. In the severe and late stages of progressive dementia, when so little is coming back from the person and there are few signs of verbal understanding, caregivers can find themselves reducing verbal interactions to a minimum. It is important to continue speaking to your relative, despite his inability to respond to or acknowledge your efforts much of the time. You want to prevent your family member's withdrawal into himself as long as you can.

Comment on what is happening in the here and now, as you provide daily care for him, or do simple things together. Continue to offer interaction and simple conversation, even though it will be one-sided. Smile and express affection often. It is likely that these caring messages *will* be understood!

## Use Touch Judiciously

Touch can be one of your main means of communicating with your family member when verbal communication is no longer effective. A gentle, reassuring pat on the arm, a hug, or a kiss tell him that he is loved and that you continue to be there for him. Holding the individual's hand can be reassuring and provide a sense of security. Use touch frequently, especially if your family member seems to respond positively to this mode of communication.

Keep in mind, though, that for some people with severe dementia, an unexpected touch, or reaching toward them can be frightening and cause anxiety or even a hostile reaction (such as striking out) because they are no longer able to interpret their environment. For example, your relative may no longer be able to recognize you or other family members as people he knows and who care for him. To lessen the chances of a negative reaction from the person with severe dementia, be sure that your relative can see you as you approach and reach out to him. Speak calmly and gently and offer a warm smile as you make contact. Use reassuring words, along with gentle touch.

## Utilize Nonverbal Communication

Even when words themselves are no longer understood, the person with severe dementia may still be able to understand gestures, pictures, and other nonverbal cues. To increase the chances that your family member will understand your messages, use these communication strategies (along with speech) as much as possible. In addition to the importance of touch (discussed above), show him, gesture, or demonstrate what it is you want him to understand. For example, your relative who does not respond when you ask him if he wants some juice may reach for and take a cup of juice if it is offered to him. He may understand about whom you are speaking if he is shown a photograph of a close family member. He may understand that you need to help him put his shirt on if you hold the item out to him as you talk about getting dressed. If you've been employing these communication methods throughout earlier phases of his illness, these skills will be especially helpful to you now. Remember that the purpose of using as many communication channels as possible is to help your loved one maintain contact with his environment and his family as long as he can.

## Assume That Your Family Member Comprehends

In this chapter, we have emphasized the profound erosion of the ability to understand verbal messages that occurs in dementia's later stages. Nevertheless, it is difficult to know for certain what messages are and are not getting through. For this reason, it continues to be very important to be wary of saying things in your relative's presence that you would not want him to hear. The best rule of thumb is to *assume* that your family member might be understanding what is said, and to discuss matters that you do not wish him to hear when he is not present. Keeping this in mind will help you remember your loved one's humanity and personhood despite his debilitating illness and the sadness you feel because he has lost so much of himself.

## Look for Signs of Comfort or Discomfort

Although in dementia's severe and final stages your relative will no longer be able to tell you that he has pain, feels ill, is frightened, or is quite comfortable, these feelings will be communicated in other ways. If he makes sounds or speaks some words, his tone of voice (fearful? angry? in distress?) will give you clues. His body postures and movements will also communicate how he is feeling. Read his body language. Does he appear calm, quiet, and restful or is he "fussing" with his clothing or moving restlessly? Facial expression, though greatly reduced in advanced dementia, may also give you a hint as to what is going on. For example, does your relative wince in pain if food is placed in his mouth, suggesting that a denture may be rubbing, or a tooth may need attention? Does his facial expression show pain when urinating, indicating a possible infection?

Other gestures will communicate to you as well. Does he clutch his side or his stomach and push food away when he has been a good eater up to this time? Does he indicate shoulder discomfort when being dressed? All of these communications suggest that examination by an appropriate health care specialist may be in order.

At the same time, your relative's positive feelings will be communicated nonverbally as well. If he has a relaxed body posture, appears calm and contented, or gives you a smile, these are indications that he is most probably comfortable. If he is cooperative as you provide care for basic needs such as dressing, bathing, and feeding, that is also a sign that he is not experiencing distress. All of these nonverbal cues are your relative's way of communicating with you when he no longer has the words to use. Be alert to his nonverbal messages.

## Encourage Attempts to Communicate

Not all individuals in the severe stages of dementia are nonverbal. You'll want to continue to reinforce those efforts your loved one makes to have verbal contact with you. If he attempts to speak, even with fragments of phrases and jargon, you may be able to figure out enough of the message to understand the gist of what he is trying to tell you. Don't simply ignore these seemingly meaningless speech attempts, but respond to them with verbal reassurance and an effort to understand them.

## Provide Other Types of Stimulation

Listening to favorite or well-loved music or tapes of familiar songs, or engaging in some simple, gentle exercises with you may still give pleasure to the person with severe dementia. If your relative appears to respond to these types of stimulation, continue to make them available to him. Let his behavior be a guide. Does familiar music seem to calm him and reduce restless behavior? Does he appear to enjoy the tactile stimulation of having something to touch or hold in his hand? If so, see that he has such items available. You may come up with other ideas for providing listening, looking, or touching experiences for your family member.

# Chapter 10

# Communicating with Family and Friends

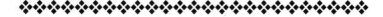

Most people with dementia and their main caregiver do not live in isolation. Family and friends are an important part of their lives. This social network is a potentially valuable support resource as you struggle with the daily demands of this devastating illness. At the same time, family and close friends will also be affected by the dementia. It will be important to both you and your impaired family member to maintain communication ties with family and close friends. Coping with the multiple challenges and daily stresses presented by a family member's progressive dementing illness is difficult enough even with the support of others to assist you. With such support, however, the task is made easier and more manageable. Knowing that you are not "in this alone" can give a big lift to your spirits.

This chapter, then, is about keeping communication channels open within the larger circle of your family and friends. They will need to understand how dementia affects memory, the ability to learn new information, judgment, and behavior as you have come to understand these things. They will want to know how they can help and how to respond to your relative's broken communication attempts, memory lapses, and sometimes difficult behaviors. On the other hand, you will need to learn how your loved one's dementia is affecting the other members of the family and your group of close friends. They will grieve along with you for lost abilities and for the person they no longer know.

## Why Involve Family and Friends Early?

Once a diagnosis of Alzheimer's disease has been made, you will need to plan to communicate this information to other people close to you and your family member. Out of fear, embarrassment, or concern that once others know they will stay away or treat your loved one differently, you may be tempted not to share the upsetting news. There are many good reasons, however, for setting these feelings aside and confiding in your close family and good friends.

First, if there has been sufficient personality change and memory impairment in your relative to warrant a diagnosis of Alzheimer's disease, others have also noted that something is wrong. Sharing the diagnosis with important others will help them to understand some of the changes they have observed in your relative. Getting family members involved early in this way can help them to deal with some of their own fears and/or lack of knowledge about dementing illness. You can talk together about ways of dealing with the illness in as positive a way as possible before feelings are hurt and nerves are frayed.

Second, your own ability to care for your family member depends on your obtaining regular breaks from the daily stresses of caregiving. If you are to continue to care for the person with dementia, you'll need to maintain your physical and mental health. Even when dementia is mild and your relative is still functioning relatively independently, you'll need time to yourself occasionally to shop, take care of personal business, enjoy a favorite hobby, have lunch with a good friend, or rest and relax. Close friends and family may be able to provide these occasional respite breaks that are so important not just for you, but for your relative.

Third, spending time with other people, especially in the early and middle stages of dementia, is good for the memory-impaired person. Seeing other familiar people and having the opportunity to participate in a variety of activities can be enjoyable and provide stimulation for him.

Finally, if family and friends can participate in caregiving and share responsibilities even in small ways, they will be helped to cope with their grieving over the losses the memory-impaired person is experiencing. It is important to realize that we don't just grieve for someone we care about when he or she actually dies. We grieve on an ongoing basis for the loss of the personality, talents, and other gifts that dementing illness takes away. It is an *unselfish act* on your part to allow others to help.

## What If Help Isn't Forthcoming?

At some times, and in some individual circumstances, families and friends don't come forth on their own with offers of assistance. This can leave the primary caring person feeling abandoned and angry. If this is true in your particular situation, it will help you to understand some of the reasons why others may not be helping. The following is a list of possible reasons why family and close friends are not sharing the work of providing care. The items on this list can be viewed as *barriers* to communication. Do any of these explanations apply in your situation? If so, decide which barriers you might be able to change, or eliminate. Is education of family and friends what is called for? Does their lack of assistance have anything to do with how you view the situation? Look at the list carefully. Think about how you might improve family communication related to the dementing illness. How can you let others know the types of assistance you would find helpful?

1. Family members might not understand how Alzheimer's disease works and the effects it has on the impaired person as well as on the main caregiver.

2. You might be trying to "protect" family and friends from the knowledge that your relative has a progressive dementing illness, not wanting to "burden" them or embarrass the memory-impaired person. When others ask about how things are going, do you downplay the problems and the stress you feel?

3. Others might be frightened by the disease, or of your family member's changed behavior, or of what he might do if they offer to spend some time with him. They may feel that they could not cope with a memory-impaired person. Some of the individual's anger outbursts and accusations (if such have occurred) might have been directed at them.

4. Other family members, especially those particularly close to the memory-impaired person, may be having a

difficult time accepting the diagnosis that the condition is irreversible and progressive. Their way of coping at the moment is to deny the reality of the situation. At the same time, they may feel sad and angry because of the impaired person's difficulties.

5. Family and friends may not know what specific kinds of help you would find most useful, even though they could provide certain types of assistance.

6. Because the person with Alzheimer's disease can appear so physically well, especially in the early to middle phases of the illness, others may not appreciate that caring for someone who is not yet physically impaired is complicated and demanding. They may not understand that you could use help *now* in your caregiving job.

7. Others may be afraid of overcommitting themselves and disrupting their own family life if they offer help. They may not realize that even occasional assistance in a small way or with a small task would be helpful.

8. Other members of the family may not feel as much responsibility to help because they are less close to the person with dementia than you are.

9. Others may not know *how* to offer their assistance, even though they would like to do so. They may be concerned about insulting you or implying that you're not doing an adequate job as the main caregiver. They may also be concerned, especially early in the disease, that their offers of help will be taken as implying that the memory-impaired person is incapable of doing anything for himself.

10. Others may sense that you feel no one else knows your relative, his habits, and his needs as well as you do. They may believe that it would be "interfering" if they offered help, that you would feel that other caregivers or respite providers couldn't "measure up" to your level of care and concern for your relative.

# Breaking Down the Barriers: Ways of Involving Family and Friends

It is sometimes difficult to ask for assistance, especially when you know that potential helpers also lead busy, often hectic lives. Nevertheless, one of the communication skills you must foster is the ability to ask for assistance if potential help is available. You owe it to yourself and to your relative with dementia to do this. Keep in mind that people are often glad to help when asked, even though they might not offer assistance on their own. You may find some of the suggestions offered below useful in communicating with family and close friends.

## Educate Others About Dementia

Once others understand the nature of progressive dementing illness, and the responsibilities and stresses it can place on the main caregiver, they may be more receptive to assisting. There are some excellent books about dementia listed in Chapter 17. They can be suggested to family and friends for background reading. Share with close others what you have learned from health care professionals about the disease and about your relative's particular situation. If you feel that you might not communicate the information as effectively or completely as a health care professional would, arrange a meeting between your relative's physician (or other appropriate professional) and close members of the family.

If your circumstances permit, see if you can have your impaired relative spend a few days or a week with a close member of the family. This might be especially helpful if family members appear to be denying the severity of your relative's impairments. They may need to see for themselves what you are coping with on a daily basis.

If you are attending an Alzheimer's support group (more about support groups later), invite other members of the family or a close friend to join you from time to time. Educating other family members and friends about dementia can be an important first step in sharing the caregiving.

## Share Effective Communication Techniques

You will want to share with others who are spending time with your relative on a regular basis some of the communication techniques that you have found to be effective. You can describe for them what works in getting through to the affected person, and what strategies aid him in expressing himself. Give them concrete examples, or better yet, model for them how you communicate with your family member. Hopefully, you'll share some of the ideas suggested in this book with other family members and friends.

## Maintain Contacts Between the Person with Dementia and Others

Encourage short visits from family and close friends. Explain to them why these visits are important to the person with dementia. Maintain social activities with family and friends as long as you can, even though you may have to change the types of activities and the length of your family member's participation as his dementia worsens.

## Be Specific About What is Needed

When you seek assistance from a member of the family, a neighbor, or a friend, be clear and specific about what you need. Open-ended requests for help may make these potential care providers uneasy. They may be concerned about becoming too involved, or overcommitting their time. If what you need is someone to come in and keep your relative company for 2 hours once a week, ask for that. If it would be helpful to have the neighbors pick up milk and bread when they are grocery shopping because you are unable to get away on a particular day, approach them with that request.

## Consider a Family Meeting

In some circumstances, it might be helpful to arrange a family meeting fairly early after a diagnosis of dementia has been made, and to schedule meetings of the close relatives at regular intervals over time. The main purpose of such meetings would be to communicate your current needs for assistance and your relative's needs for companionship and stimulation, and to come up with a plan for sharing caregiving responsibilities. Another reason for meeting together would be to share information with the family about your relative's current status and results of recent testing or medical evaluations.

Which family members should attend such meetings is an individual decision and depends on individual circumstances. In some situations you might want to include close friends as well as members of the close family. You will want to think carefully about whether to include children or the memory-impaired person himself. In some cases including the person with dementia helps him to see that others care and are concerned about him.

In preparing for such a family meeting, if you decide to plan one, there are some questions you need to ask yourself.

1. What do you want this particular meeting to achieve?

2. Are there specific types of assistance you need, or a particular problem to work through?

3. Are there decisions that need to be made at this time?

4. What do you want the outcome of the meeting to be?

There are questions about the details of the meeting to be worked out as well. When and where do you want the meeting to take place? Do you want to ask someone to conduct, or facilitate, the meeting? It could be you the caregiver, another member of the family, or perhaps a trusted outside person such as your minister, priest, or rabbi. Do you want someone to take notes at the meeting, and summarize them for those present? It can be helpful to have a written plan, especially if the purpose of the meeting is to come up with ways to share current caregiving responsibilities.

## Be Flexible

Over the course of a dementing illness, the circumstances and responsibilities of different members of your support system may change. Individuals who were able to provide respite for you and outings for your affected relative may now find that they have increased family or work responsibilities. Others may be temporarily unable to help because of their own health problems. On the other hand, some family members who had little time to contribute earlier may be a great source of support to you now. You need to manage these changes in your close support system with flexibility and understanding. Let people know that you realize circumstances have changed and that you have appreciated their assistance. They may be able to step in at some future time and be of help.

# Communicating with Children about Dementia

If there are children in the family who are affected by your relative's dementing illness, you will want to give their needs and their reactions to the illness some special attention. Children may be perplexed and upset by the changes they see in a beloved parent or grandparent. They may not understand why so much of your time is now taken up with the care of your family member. They may withdraw from their friends because they are embarrassed by the affected person's behavior.

On the other hand, children are resilient. They will respond positively to an explanation of the disease and its effects. Children can understand what has happened to Grandpa or Grandma if you gear your explanation to their level of comprehension and vocabulary. Take time to talk with your children, to explain the disease, and to let them express their feelings. Even if they do not express their concerns, children may blame themselves for what is occurring unless they are given other explanations. It's important that they understand that their relative has an illness, that the illness isn't "catching," and that nothing they have done has caused the affected person to become ill. Younger children may need special reassurance that you will not become ill.

Children will quickly pick up on your communication strategies in talking with the memory-impaired person, including your tone of voice. Your demonstrations of positive, gentle, and patient communication approaches with your relative will be adopted by them. As they see you treating the memory-impaired person with respect and consideration, they will do the same. Another positive aspect of having children in the environment is that they are often more accepting of the behaviors of someone with dementia (forgetfulness, word-finding problems, misnaming items) than are adults. Young children and frail elderly adults can be wonderful companions to one another.

Incorporate the children in your household in your interactions with your relative and involve them in doing small things for the memory-impaired person. Children want to be helpful, and they can thrive on small amounts of responsibility. At the same time, don't overburden them with the care of your family member. Be sensitive to their need for time to be their own person. You don't want to rely on them too much for help.

In the list of resources in Chapter 17, there are several books on dementia written for children and some written for adolescents. If the children in your family are of reading age, you might want to obtain one or more of these books. If you live in a city or town that has a local Alzheimer's Association chapter (see Chapter 17 — Resources), they may have the books available on a loan basis. The Alzheimer's Association has published a brochure on dementia especially for teenagers. This is available at no cost from the association or one of its local chapters. Some Alzheimer's Association chapters have support groups especially for young children and adolescents.

# Chapter 11

# Other Sources of Support and Communication

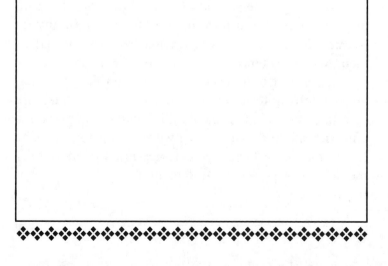

For a variety of reasons, it is not always possible to count on support from family and friends or to change family circumstances. When such support and opportunities for communication are not available, other resources must be found. You need help in caring for your relative whether or not there is family to assist, for no one, no matter how capable or how strong, can bear the burden of caring for a person with such a devastating chronic illness alone. Consider the following possibilities as you investigate ways of sharing your caregiving and finding support for yourself.

## Support Groups

Some of the best sources of information on ways to cope with dementing illness are caregiver support groups. In a supportive and accepting group setting, caregivers share their concerns and feelings with others who understand the challenges of caring for a person with dementia because they have been there themselves. They also share solutions to problems that arise in the day-to-day care of their relatives and information about community resources. Some group meetings may be educational in focus, with speakers on different topics related to dementia, such as nutrition, legal issues, community resources, and caregiving techniques. Usually support groups are facilitated by an individual familiar with group processes and with methods for dealing with sensitive issues. The leader may be a health care professional or the family member of a person with dementia.

Because public awareness of Alzheimer's disease has greatly increased in the last few years, caregiver support groups are much more numerous and available than they were even 5 years ago. You can obtain information about support groups in your area from the local chapter of the Alzheimer's Association, or from the national office of the Alzheimer's Association (the address and phone number of the national office are listed under resources in Chapter 17). Your local hospital may also sponsor such support groups for caregivers of dementia-afflicted people. Most support groups for dementia caregivers are open to the public and free of charge. Some may charge a small fee for certain educational programs.

Consider attending a caregiver support group. It may be the best thing you do for yourself. Support groups provide an opportunity for you to communicate with others who understand. You can share your feelings of frustration and exhaustion or of accomplishment and satisfaction with understanding and sympathetic listeners. You will find an atmosphere of acceptance and confidentiality. Participating in a support group will also help you gain self-confidence. You'll feel that you are more in control of your life. As you gain knowledge about the disease, begin to prepare for the future, and share problem-solving techniques, you will feel more in control of your situation. If your particular circumstances make it impossible to attend a support group, some Alzheimer's Association chapters have a telephone support network.

## Church-Related Resources

If you are affiliated with a church or a synagogue, look into the possibility of obtaining some support from that resource. Talk to your pastor, minister, or rabbi and explain your relative's illness. Let this individual know what your needs and concerns are. Many congregations have volunteers who will provide occasional companionship to their frail elderly members and at the same time offer you some welcome respite. Some have day care programs for memory-impaired adults, or other activities that can be a source of stimulation and involvement for your relative.

## Day Care and Respite Programs

Increasingly, community hospitals and other private and nonprofit organizations offer services for dementia caregivers. Among such services are adult day care programs, respite programs, and many kinds of in-home assistance. Adult day care programs offer a variety of activities for the person with dementia, while at the same time providing valuable relief for the caregiver.

Formal respite services and programs may include a range of options. These vary from a few hours of in-home companionship for the memory-impaired person while the caregiver takes some time off, to longer stays for the affected individual in a care facility to provide extended respite for the caregiver. Respite services can be arranged through home health agencies, adult family homes or foster homes, and residential care facilities.

**Other Sources of Support and Communication**

Chapter 14 further explores the topic of how to obtain needed caregiving help and offers suggestions for communicating with providers of respite, day care, and other services.

# Chapter 12

# Communicating with Health Care Professionals

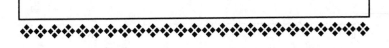

In your role as a primary caregiver for someone with a dementing illness, you've taken on many important functions. One of these functions is communicating with those individuals who provide health care and other formal services to your family member. As the caring person for someone whose memory, communication skills, and other cognitive abilities are declining, you will need to assume the role of "health care consumer/advocate" for him. This chapter offers some suggestions for getting the most out of these important interactions with health care professionals, such as physicians, nurses, therapists, and others.

## Your Role as Advocate

Even in the early stages of progressive dementia, when communication skills are still relatively intact, you as the caring family member will find yourself acting as advocate for your relative. If a diagnosis of probable Alzheimer's disease has not yet been made, but you suspect that something is wrong with your loved one, convincing him to see a physician may be difficult. The person may deny that he is having any problems with memory or with performing on the job. You may find yourself facing the brunt of your family member's anger for suggesting a visit to the doctor.

On the other hand, your loved one may sense that something is "not quite right," and want to seek some answers. In either case, you will need to persist in seeing that a thorough medical workup is completed and some answers obtained if you are convinced that your relative needs a medical evaluation. If your family physician does not appear to be knowledgeable about or interested in dementing illnesses (and many are not), you may want to request a referral to a *neurologist,* a medical specialist in diagnosing and treating diseases of the brain and nervous system. In many larger cities, special dementia evaluation clinics can be found where teams of specialists in dementia can assist you.

As the dementing illness progresses, you will find yourself advocating for your family member to assure that appropriate services are available to him. These services may include ongoing medical and dental care, periodic evaluations of memory, learning, and judgment functions to determine appropriate management strategies, speech and language evaluations, assessments of hearing functions, and therapies if appropriate.

## Suggestions for Communicating with Health Care Professionals

Your interactions with the variety of health care professionals you will meet can be positive and fruitful if you make use of some of the communication tips offered below. You should leave such visits with the feeling that your questions have been answered, that the information you sought was provided, and that your concerns have been addressed. Look over these suggestions and adopt those that seem most useful to you. They can serve as a guide for all of your contacts with health care personnel.

## Prepare for Visits Beforehand

The time you spend preparing for appointments before the visit can pay great dividends. The following list of suggestions will help you to get ready for medical appointments so that you get the most out of them.

1. *Do some background reading.* If the diagnosis of dementia is still in question, you may want to do some background reading, especially before the first medical evaluation appointment. Select one or two references from the resources listed in Chapter 17. Request some of the excellent pamphlets and brochures available through such organizations as the Alzheimer's Association, the American Association of Retired Persons (AARP), or the U.S. Government's Department of Veterans Affairs (formerly the Veterans Administration) if your family member is a veteran. Many of these resources are provided without cost. The more you can educate yourself about dementing illness, the better you'll understand some of the medical terms and other information discussed at the appointment.

2. *Prepare a list of specific questions* and concerns beforehand, and write them down. You might want to purchase a small notebook in which you can jot down your questions as they occur to you. In this way, you're always preparing for the next scheduled visit. Before the visit, go over your notes and make a list of those specific points you want to discuss. Keep in mind that it is easier for health care personnel to respond to your questions than to guess what might be on your mind or to anticipate your particular needs.

Don't think that you're being presumptuous or hostile in asking questions. Remind yourself that one of the health care team's major responsibilities is to answer your questions and concerns. Health care providers will appreciate the fact that you have come to the visit well prepared. Being armed with a list of questions will help you to communicate clearly and will serve to make the best use of everyone's time, including yours.

3. *Have a list of all medications that your relative is currently taking.* Include both prescription and nonprescription drugs.

4. Health care personnel may also want to know how much tobacco, alcohol, and caffeine-containing substances (coffee, tea, chocolate) your family member uses.

5. *Write down the impaired person's typical or usual daily schedule.* Include information about activities that he enjoys, rest periods, mealtimes, and the like.

6. *Make a list of any problems that have come up since the last visit.* Include some information about how frequently these problems occur and the circumstances that seem to trigger problem behaviors or concerns.

7. *Include some questions and information about how you are doing!* It is easy to focus only on your family member and to neglect concerns about yourself. Yet information about the stresses you are experiencing and how you view your own physical health and well-being is very important to health care providers. Dementia care involves not just treating the affected person but his caregiver as well.

This information can also be kept in the notebook in which you've jotted down your questions. If you date your notes, the book becomes a daily diary of your relative's needs and how he is doing, as well as of your needs and concerns.

8. *Plan so that enough time is allowed for the visit.* If you have a number of items to discuss or questions to ask, let the individual who schedules appointments know that you would like to have more time at the next visit.

9. *Remember to organize any assistance that you'll need on the day of the appointment,* such as transportation or help with getting your relative ready for the visit. Be sure to do this well ahead of time.

10. *Consider scheduling a conference without your impaired family member present* occasionally, so that you can discuss your concerns more openly.

## Communicate Clearly and Effectively

There are a number of things you can do to increase the chances that good communication occurs during visits with health care providers. Because you have prepared for the visit beforehand, you have already done a great deal to assure that you and the health care team *can* communicate effectively. Here are some additional suggestions.

1. *Bring your written notes or notebook with you* to the visit, including your list of questions. In some circumstances, you might want to bring your relative's actual medicines with you as well (especially if you are seeing a new health care provider for the first time).

2. *Be prepared to take some notes* during the visit. You will want to write down specific suggestions and recommendations made so that you will remember them accurately. Consider bringing another family member or good friend with you, not only for support, but to take notes so that you can listen and concentrate on the information being provided.

3. *Repeat back to the health care provider,* in your own words, what you think has just been said to you. This is a good communication technique to develop and to get in the habit of using. It gives the health care professional the chance to immediately clear up any misunderstanding or confusion that may have occurred. You should also let the individual know when you haven't understood an explanation or some medical terms that have been used. Remember that members of the health care team *need* this kind of feedback if they are to do the best job possible for you and your loved one. They will appreciate your efforts to see that clear communication takes place.

4. *Ask questions about any new treatment or drug being recommended.* Specifically, ask about the potential benefits and risks or possible side effects of such treatments. You need this information to make informed decisions when the choice of a treatment is left up to you. You will also need to watch for potential side effects of new medications. Other questions related to medications or treatments include: Are there any other treatments available? What are the benefits and risks of such alternative treatments? Should the medication *not* be taken with any other medicines, foods, or beverages (such as alcohol)? In asking such questions you are being a wise and respon-

sible health care consumer advocate for your impaired relative who cannot ask these questions for himself.

5. *Ask the various health care team members what kind of information is helpful to them.* What do they need to know about your impaired family member? What types of information about your caregiving routines and schedule would be helpful in treating the person with dementia and providing you with support? This will help you prepare for the next visit.

6. *Ask about follow-up plans.* How often do various members of the dementia care team need to see your impaired relative? When do they want you to check back with them? If you are dealing with a health care team rather than an individual, ask if the team can designate one person whom you can call with questions or concerns. This will be helpful to you and reduce unnecessary communications.

7. *Tell the team or health care practitioner what specific kinds of help you need.* Have you reached the point in your family member's illness where you need assistance with his day-to-day care? Do you need more information and ideas about how to manage a particular dementia-related problem, such as communication difficulties, wandering, or sleeping problems? Are you looking for a caregiver support group? Is occasional respite from caregiving what you need most? Are you experiencing health problems of your own that need attention? Are you feeling the need to consider alternative care for your relative?

The team or individual you've consulted should be able to refer you to sources of assistance for your current needs, even if they cannot provide the help themselves. But first, you must let health care providers know what your needs are! Remember that they can learn from your experience in their efforts to help other dementia caregivers. As a consumer of dementia-related services, keep in mind that you are a teaching member of the team.

## Follow Through on Suggestions and Recommendations

Continued communication with the health care team between scheduled visits assures that important information about your relative and his health status is shared in a timely manner. *Call and report any sudden changes in the impaired person's symptoms or behavior promptly* to the designated team member, especially if a new medication has been recently started. If you find that you are not able to carry out a particular recommendation made by the health care provider on a recent visit, let the provider know this as soon as possible. If a particular task is difficult for you to manage, other ways to provide you with appropriate assistance can be suggested. Don't be hesitant to share that a caregiving task is too hard for you.

If you have some new care ideas you think you'd like to try, especially if they involve nonprescription medicines or an advertised "new treatment" for dementing illness, it would be wise to first speak with your relative's physician or another appropriate member of the dementia team. Discuss possible side effects of the over-the-counter drug with the physician.

# Have Realistic Expectations

Because your relationship with the health care team is such a close and ongoing one, there may be times when you feel disappointment, anger, and frustration that team members cannot offer you and your impaired family member a cure for this terrible disease. Experiencing these feelings is normal, especially early in the illness, or if you and your relative have just completed an initial dementia evaluation. You may still need more time to take in the news that your loved one has a progressive, debilitating illness for which there is presently no known cure.

Nevertheless, you and the health care team will need to work together to provide your family member with the best possible care. Communicating clearly and effectively with each other will depend on your gradually coming to accept that Alzheimer's disease is a progressive and irreversible condition. Despite the fact that no one can halt the progress of the disease, the health care team can offer help in managing some of the problems that arise and can continue to support you in your caregiving efforts. Realistic expectations on your part will not necessarily occur overnight, but through ongoing communication with health care providers, mutual understanding and appropriate expectations will develop.

# When You're Not Satisfied

Despite your best efforts to communicate and a realistic perspective on dementing illness, you may feel unhappy or dissatisfied with the physician who is caring for your memory-impaired relative. You may feel that you and your family member are not getting the help you need. You may feel that your concerns are not being taken seriously. You may be feeling frustrated that your questions are not being answered.

Physicians differ widely in their ability to deal well with the complex needs of the person with dementia and with his caregiver, despite the fact that they may be very competent medical care providers. There can be many reasons why this is so. A particular physician may not fully understand the nature of dementing illness, or may not have had much experience in working with caregivers of people with dementia. The physician may be too busy to provide the amount of time needed to deal with a difficult and ongoing situation or feel that "nothing can be done" once the diagnosis of dementia has been made.

If you are dissatisfied with your relationship with your family member's physician, *look for alternatives.* You and your relative deserve and need an ongoing relationship with a health care provider or team that is knowledgeable about dementia. You need health care practitioners who can provide treatment and guidance over the course of this long, progressive disease. You deserve to have your problems and concerns taken seriously and to have assistance in working out a plan to address those problems.

# Chapter 13

# Communicating with Legal and Financial Advisers

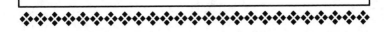

Dementing illness eventually diminishes the ability to manage one's financial and legal affairs. At some point in the course of the disease, the affected person becomes unable to make reasonable decisions involving money management and unable to plan for the future. He will forget to pay bills, or not recall those that have been paid. The impaired person will be unable to remember where important financial and legal documents are kept. He may hide these papers in difficult-to-find places, especially if the disease makes him suspicious that others are after his money. Balancing a checkbook becomes an impossible task. He may be talked into unwise purchases as judgment diminishes. Furthermore, because of memory loss and communication difficulties, he will eventually become unable to let others know his wishes regarding important decisions about his health care and about who will inherit his assets when he dies.

At the same time, having adequate financial resources, or at least making finances stretch as far as they can is crucial over the long-term. Progressive dementing illness, because it can continue over a long period of time, will use up a large share of these resources. Care needs will increase with time, including in many situations, the need to pay for outside help and other professional services or to place the individual in a care facility. Most health care insurance plans, including Medicare, do not pay for the day-to-day expenses associated with dementia care.

## How Do These Issues Affect the Caregiver?

What do these legal and financial realities mean to you as the caregiver of a person with dementia? It is likely that sooner or later you will be taking over the management of your relative's financial affairs. If you are the spouse of an impaired person, you will be concerned about not only providing adequately for your relative but looking after your own future financial needs as well. You will want to see that a decent standard of living is maintained for yourself and for your children, if children are involved. If another member of the family, or a close friend, is managing the affected person's legal and money matters, you will need to communicate with that individual about these issues.

You may also find yourself in the position of making important health care decisions, especially in the severe to final stages of the illness. Such decisions can involve whether to place a feeding tube if the person with dementia stops eating, whether he should undergo a particular surgery, or whether he should be placed on a ventilator (artificial breathing machine) if he stops breathing. To make these types of decisions for another person when he is not capable of making them for himself, you need a legal designation to do so, such as *durable power of attorney for health care* or *guardianship.*

## Durable Power of Attorney for Health Care

If you are given durable power of attorney for health care for another person it means that the individual has designated you to make health care decisions for him should he not, in the future, be able to make such decisions for himself. These wishes are put down in writing, in a legal document called a *durable power of attorney for health care.* At the time such a designation is made, however, the person must have the judgment and understanding to make such a decision. He must understand what he is doing by signing the document. That is, he must be *competent* to do so. This is an important reason for discussing health care wishes with your family member *as soon as possible*. Some states do not recognize durable power of attorney. You should check with an attorney knowledgeable in these matters or with the local chapter of the Alzheimer's Association to determine whether your state recognizes durable power of attorney.

## Guardianship

To be granted *guardianship* of another person, you must go through a formal legal process. The impaired person's inability to care for himself and to make decisions must be demonstrated to the satisfaction of the court hearing the guardianship petition. Levels of guardianship, from limited to full guardianship, also vary from state to state and may be called by different names. An attorney can help clarify guardianship issues for you.

Dealing with these difficult financial, legal, and ethical questions can be stressful for you, for other members of the family, and for the person with dementia. They are complex issues that will require you to understand perhaps unfamiliar legal and medical terms. The following suggestions are offered as a starting place. They will not provide all of the answers you need, but they should help you ask the right questions and communicate more effectively with those professionals who can help you plan for the future.

# Gather Information

Communicating clearly with lawyers, counselors, and other advisers begins with having as much information in hand as possible about your family member's financial and legal affairs before you meet with the person who is advising you. If you have not previously been communicating with your relative about such matters, this can be a difficult task. People often don't like to talk about money or health care decisions with others. They consider it their private and personal business.

If suspiciousness is part of the dementia picture, the task of gathering this information can be made even more difficult. There is also the issue of implying (often with good reason!) that the person with the dementing illness is no longer capable of dealing with money and money matters. This can be a blow to his already fragile self-esteem. It is frequently the case that elderly spouses, especially wives, have left legal and money matters up to their husbands and have not been involved in dealing with family financial concerns. Suddenly, these wives find themselves changing roles with their husbands and becoming the family financial manager. If this is the situation in which you find yourself, you need to start learning as much as you can about your relative's and the family's financial status as soon as possible.

## Assets

A good place to start educating yourself about financial matters is to take stock of the impaired person's or the family's assets.

1. Begin by gathering such information as the location and account numbers of various bank accounts, both checking and savings.
2. Determine whether there are any assets such as stocks and bonds, insurance policies, retirement accounts, and the like.
3. Is there current income available, such as social security and/or retirement payments?
4. Do other financial assets such as rental property or valuable personal collections exist?

### Expenses

After taking stock of your financial resources, you'll need to look at current and anticipated expenses.

1. What are your relative's (and yours if appropriate to include) current ongoing expenses for shelter, food, medicines, and other items?
2. Are there debts such as a home mortgage or outstanding personal loans?
3. What future (near and long-term) expenses can be anticipated?

If you have already selected a financial adviser, be it another family member or someone else, ask them what other kinds of information they would like to have available for an initial visit, such as income tax returns, bank statements, or wills.

## Assume Control Tactfully

Taking over the management of your family member's financial affairs as tactfully as possible can be a challenge. The process may begin gradually, as you assist the impaired person in paying bills. You may in time take over managing the checkbook and monitoring expenditures. At an appropriate time (preferably sooner than later) you will need to determine where your relative keeps important papers relating to financial and legal matters.

Remember that the onset of dementia is a gradual process and that the affected person may retain some ability to specify his wishes and participate in decision making for a long time. Letting your relative feel that he is included in decisions will help things to go more smoothly. Keep in mind that a primary goal of dementia care is to allow the impaired person to keep as much control over his life and his affairs as is reasonably possible.

## Seek the Advice of Others

If you need assistance in choosing someone to help you, there are several possibilities.

1. If you happen to have a family lawyer already, start with that person.
2. You might ask other family members and friends if they know of someone who is knowledgeable and trustworthy and if they have had personal experience in dealing with that person.
3. You can obtain the names of lawyers who specialize in assisting families in your situation from the local Bar Association's Attorney Referral Service.
4. Local Senior Centers and other agencies often can suggest lawyers or other competent advisers.

5. You might also consider asking your local banker or someone else you trust if they can recommend someone.
6. Members of dementia support groups can be a valuable source of information on where to seek legal and financial advice.

The important thing is to select someone who has the expertise to help you manage current financial matters and to plan for the future. This person should also be someone you can work with comfortably.

## Begin Early

You may be tempted to postpone dealing with these vital financial concerns. It can be difficult to bring up the sensitive subject of money with an impaired relative or with other members of the family. Your motives for doing so may be questioned. Bringing up financial matters may upset the person with dementia and trigger arguments and accusations.

Nevertheless, it is crucial that you begin communicating about these issues as early in the course of the dementing illness as possible. Your relative may, before memory loss becomes severe, be able to show you where important papers are located and to explain what assets and financial obligations exist. He may be able to play a role in choosing a financial adviser and in making other important money-related decisions. Remember that you will want to talk about financial and legal issues while your relative still has the communication skills to participate in such a dialogue, if this is possible. Approach the task, if your situation permits, from the point of view that you and your family member are partners in doing this early planning for the future.

# Plan for Future Needs

Another reason for beginning the process of educating yourself about your relative's and the family's financial situation early is that it will help you to plan wisely for future needs. It may be difficult to imagine expensive future care needs when your relative is still communicating well and is able to care for himself in most ways. With time, however, dementia-related financial obligations will become greater. The earlier you can begin planning for these future expenses, the more likely it is that resources will stretch further. For example, the interest or dividends earned by placing your family member's assets in a place that will include the right balance of financial risk and financial return can add substantially to future available resources. Seek expert advice *early* in planning for the future.

# Communicate with the Family

In many families, dementia caregiving is a shared responsibility. In the same way, responsibility for financial decision making may be shared among family members. Family meetings to deal with these concerns can be an excellent communication tool for some families. The meetings may be used to discuss and weigh financial planning options, to come to agreement on ways to share the monetary costs of caring for the person with dementia, or to delegate responsibility for the management of the impaired person's finances. It may be that the best person to look after your family member's financial and legal matters is not the person providing most of the day-to-day care.

The meetings can also serve the purpose of keeping all close family members informed about the impaired person's financial situation. If you are the spouse of a person with progressive dementia and you have not had much previous experience in dealing with money matters, adult children may be helpful to you in making financial decisions. Occasional family meetings to discuss the subject of finances will provide an opportunity for adult children to assist.

It may be that you are the major person overseeing the management of your loved one's financial and legal affairs. If so, you will want to keep other close family members informed of the decisions you make and how the impaired person's resources are being spent. Periodic written reports of expenditures and income can save possible misunderstandings later. Communication with family about financial concerns will be easier if you keep careful records of all transactions. This will protect you and save confusion.

## Tap Other Resources

In preparing yourself to assume responsibility for legal and financial decisions, the more information you have the better. The more knowledgeable you are the better communicator you'll be with those professionals who will be assisting you.

## Books and Other Reading Material

Chapter 17 offers suggestions for reading in more detail about these complex issues. Some of the books that provide an overview of caregiving issues in dementing illness, such as *The 36 Hour Day* and *Understanding Alzheimer's Disease* would be good places to start. The Glossary in the Appendix of this book defines some of the legal terms related to decision making and competency.

## Organizations Concerned with Alzheimer's Disease and Aging

You can also obtain valuable information about seeking legal and financial planning help by writing or calling some of the organizations listed in Chapter 17, especially the Alzheimer's Association, the American Association of Retired Persons (AARP), and the U. S. Government's Department of Veterans Affairs.

For example, the Alzheimer's Association has a number of pamphlets and books available, some at no cost, that deal with legal and financial issues. The AARP has a publication available entitled *Tomorrow's Choices: Preparing Now for Future Legal, Financial, and Health Care Decisions*. Dr. Kenneth Hepburn of the Minneapolis, Minnesota, Veterans Affairs Medical Center has written a series of helpful pamphlets dealing with many aspects of coping with Alzheimer's disease, including three bro- chures concerned with legal and financial planning issues.

As you take advantage of these resources, however, keep in mind that laws vary from state to state, and that family circumstances are unique as well. It is essential for you to communicate with a person who is knowledgeable about the laws in your state and who knows or who can get to know your situation.

# Chapter 14

# Communicating with Government and Private Service Agencies

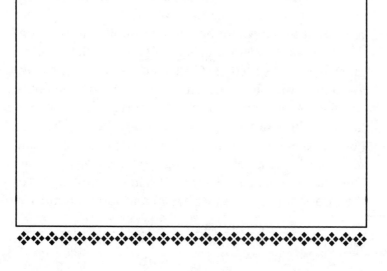

Whether or not you're currently experiencing the need for caregiving help, there will come a time when you recognize that you need assistance in caring for your relative. While some help may come from family and friends, you may find yourself seeking services from formal care providers such as governmental agencies or privately operated programs. At the very least, you need to learn about what kind of help is out there for you, if and when you should want it.

Communicating with service agencies can be frustrating and tiresome. Jokes and complaints about "bureaucracies" are commonplace. It often seems as if the amount of paperwork you are required to fill out and the array of people you have to contact makes the task of seeking assistance hardly worth the effort. Don't become discouraged at such times.

Often the best possible support for someone with a dementing illness and for the caregiver is obtained through a combination of family, friends, and caregiving agencies working together. For example, you find that you can continue to manage the increasing care needs of your relative at home where he is comfortable and less confused *because* he attends the Adult Day Health Care Program at a nearby Medical Center, and *because* you receive assistance with his care from other family members. Another caregiver in the family support group you attend describes how rested she feels and how her spirits have perked up because her relative received good respite care for 2 weeks at a local nursing care facility while she enjoyed a much needed vacation. These are examples of the informal (family and friends) and formal (paid service agencies and personnel) caregiving systems cooperating to provide good care for the person with dementia.

## Communication is the Goal

You can develop your skills in communicating effectively with agency personnel. Remember that the people you contact are there to serve you and your family member, and that they are professionals trying to do the best job that they can. They are often as frustrated with bureaucratic red tape and seemingly unreasonable regulations as you are.

Service providers do not feel good if they haven't been able to help you. By maintaining a positive and persistent attitude, you can usually get what you need and want. The following ideas will help you to be a more effective and efficient communicator when dealing with formal service providers.

## Determine What Services You Need Now

To be well prepared to ask about help that may be available, you need to first determine what kind of assistance you need. A good place to start is to *make a list of problems you are experiencing with caregiving now*. Be as specific as you can, and remember to think about yourself as well as your family member. Perhaps the impaired person's needs are being met very well at the moment, but you are experiencing fatigue and lack of companionship. As you prepare your list, you might ask yourself some of the following questions.

1. Is the impaired person's *physical* care getting to be too much for me?
2. Does my relative need some outside activity and stimulation?
3. Do we need assistance working through legal and financial issues?
4. Am I concerned about finances and paying for necessary home care?
5. Do I need someone to come into the home a few hours each week so that I can accomplish necessary business and get away on my own for a while?

## Think About Future Needs

In addition to your list of current needs for assistance, *make a list of anticipated problems and the types of help you may need in the future.* Perhaps you know that a family member who has been a big help to you will be moving away in a few months. You may see that the physical care of your impaired relative will become a greater concern in the near future. Although no one has a crystal ball through which they can see exactly what lies ahead, you should be able to give some thought to how family circumstances, your own health needs, or your relative's declining condition may call for different types of help or more frequent assistance some months from now. Actually writing down lists of problems and needs for assistance will help organize your thoughts when you are ready to make inquiries of service agencies.

## Educate Yourself About Resources

After you have spent some time thinking about your family's need for caregiving support, you're ready to start learning about what kinds of help are available in your community. Some places to start this process include your local chapter of the Alzheimer's Association or the national office of that organization; the state Area Agency on Aging; local Senior Centers; neighborhood or city-wide information and referral services emphasizing the needs of the elderly; the social work departments of hospitals; and local churches or synagogues. Family support groups can be another good place to talk with others in similar circumstances about finding help.

Look over the list of organizational resources in Chapter 17. Several of them have publications available on such issues as finding good home care, evaluating respite care, and selecting a nursing home. Many of these publications contain specific questions to ask service providers in evaluating their appropriateness for you and your family member. Several of the books listed under the references can also be helpful in guiding your decision making.

## Communicate Your Needs Clearly

Prepared with a list of your current and potential needs for specific services, and with a general idea of what types of resources are available in your community, you're now ready to do some calling. If making these kinds of calls is difficult for you, or if you feel nervous, you may want to rehearse a call with a family member or a friend, or take someone with you to visit an agency. You might want to begin with an agency that seems to have the broadest array of either direct services or of information about services. Remember that the first person with whom you speak may be a receptionist or secretary, who can only direct your call to the appropriate individual. You might initially say, on reaching an agency, "I need to speak with someone about transportation services for my relative who has dementia."

In making these calls, be prepared to be put on hold for what can seem like long periods of time. Eventually, you'll get to speak with someone who can assist you. Utilize the following suggestions in making your calls.

## Be Well Organized

Having your thoughts and notes well organized will allow you to be brief and to communicate your specific needs directly. When making phone calls about available services, you do not need to relate your relative's entire medical history or all of the details about his dementia symptoms. A brief description of your current circumstances and specific need for assistance will be enough to begin the conversation. Also, have a list of prepared questions that you will want to ask.

1. Can this particular agency provide the type of service in which you are interested?
2. Is there a cost for the service? If so, is there a sliding fee scale, depending on one's income?

3. Are there eligibility requirements for the service, such as income below a certain level, that the person be of at least a certain age, or have a specific diagnosis?
4. At what times and how frequently is the service provided? For example, Meals on Wheels may be delivered on weekdays only from 11:30 a.m. to 1:30 p.m.
5. What action on your part is necessary to obtain the service? Will you need to fill out some paper work? Is an in-person interview required? Does the agency need to meet with your impaired relative? For example, if you are seeking an adult day care program for your impaired family member, the program personnel might want to meet with him to determine whether their program would meet his needs and whether he meets their program requirements.
6. Is there a particular geographic area that is covered by the agency, and is your family member eligible?

Some of your questions may be answered without the need to ask them, but have a list of questions written out just in case.

## Keep Written Notes

You should have paper and pencil available when you begin making telephone inquiries about services. Be sure to jot down the date on which you made the call, the name or names of individuals to whom you spoke, their titles or positions, and their telephone numbers. This will make it easier for you to make those inevitable follow-up phone calls. Make a note of the specific information the person provides and ask if he has written information available that he could send you. Keeping a notebook with all of the information you gather from service agencies can help you keep your notes organized and available.

## Follow Up Promptly

Many times, an agency employee won't be able to give you a definite answer about the availability of a particular service on the first telephone call. You may be told that someone will get back to you with an answer. Don't hesitate to ask when you might be able to expect a follow-up call.

If you don't hear anything from the agency by the designated time, you should call back. Things happen in busy agencies. Names and telephone numbers get misplaced. New agency crises or concerns arise. Follow up with repeat telephone calls if you haven't received an answer, and remember not to wait too long to do this. Your persistence will pay off! Remember that you are acting as advocate for both yourself and for your impaired relative. You don't have to wait!

## Don't Let Paperwork Be a Barrier

Obtaining services from government agencies or community programs can be complicated by lots of paperwork, and/or waiting in lines in agency offices. There is usually no way to avoid this red tape. The sooner you complete the necessary forms, however, the sooner the assistance you and your family member need can be obtained. If you've received some paperwork from an agency that needs to be filled out and returned, do so promptly. If you find it difficult or annoying to complete required forms, perhaps you can get some help to complete the task from a friend, a family member, or someone who is counseling you.

## Ask for Information About Other Resources

Many times, you may be told that a particular agency can't provide the service you're requesting. When this happens, ask whether the person to whom you're speaking can suggest another agency or community resource you might try. If they respond positively, see if you can obtain the name of a person in the second agency to contact. It always helps to have the name of a particular individual to call and to be able to say that "Ms. Janet Fox of the Senior Services Division referred me to you."

## Don't Get Discouraged

Finding your way through the maze of agencies that assist people with Alzheimer's disease and their caregivers can seem overwhelming at times. You may have to try several organizations before you locate one that can provide, for example, in-home respite care that is of acceptable quality at a cost you can afford. No service is

perfect, and you may find at times that you need to com-
promise, or to look elsewhere for a particular kind of
help. Keep up your efforts to find the best available services for your relative and for yourself. It is worth the
effort to obtain that vital assistance you need to keep up
your caregiving work.

# Chapter 15

# The Relationship Between Problem Behaviors and Communication Difficulty

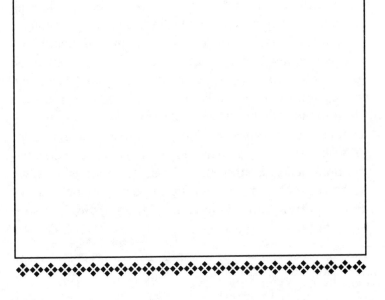

❖❖❖❖❖❖❖❖❖❖❖❖❖❖❖❖❖❖❖❖❖❖❖❖❖❖❖❖❖❖❖❖❖❖

Disruptive or disturbing behaviors frequently accompany the gradual deterioration of memory, judgment, language abilities, and personality that characterize progressive dementia. The degree to which your family member will show any of the behaviors described in this chapter will depend on both the pattern of his disease progression and on what approaches are used to prevent or manage disruptive behavior. Keep in mind that, while problem behaviors are quite common in dementing illness, not all people with dementia will show these behaviors.

## What Do We Know About Problem Behaviors in Dementia?

There is still a lot that we do not know about problem behaviors in Alzheimer's disease. For example, we don't have good information on how frequently or how commonly different troublesome behaviors occur. There is still much to be learned about what causes such problem behaviors. We do know, however, that difficult behaviors can be managed successfully. Some behaviors, such as sleeplessness and severe restlessness may be effectively managed through the judicious use of medication under the guidance of a knowledgeable physician. Other troublesome behaviors respond to preventive measures and to what are known as behavior management, or behavior modification, strategies. These techniques involve being consistent in responding to particular behaviors, and rewarding those behaviors of the impaired person that are positive and desirable.

# Communication Difficulties and Behavior

The focus of this chapter will be on the relationship between communication problems and some of the difficult behaviors you may observe in your relative. Frequently, the inability to communicate a need, desire, or source of discomfort leads to problem behaviors. Likewise, not being able to understand a spoken request or direction can result in a negative response from the impaired individual. Understanding the basis for these behaviors can be the first step in helping you reduce their occurrence and deal more effectively with them.

# Perceptions of Troublesome Behaviors

Problem behaviors, to some extent, are also "in the eye of the beholder." A particular behavior that may not be especially bothersome to you (for example, pacing or rummaging) may be very upsetting to another caregiver. That caregiver, however, may handle verbal repetitive behavior relatively easily, while you find the constant repeating of questions by the memory-impaired person particularly annoying. It's important to keep in mind that people vary in their ability to tolerate different troublesome behaviors.

# Causes of Behavior Seen in Alzheimer's Disease

It is easy to assume that problem behaviors are "caused" by the dementing illness itself, especially if you have read or have been told to expect certain behaviors at different stages of the illness. Be cautious, however, about concluding that dementia is the direct cause of changes you observe in your family member's behavior or abilities. Consider other possibilities first, such as environmental factors (noise, confusion, lots of activity), physical health factors (an infection, pain, physical discomfort), or communication factors (inability to express the need to go to the bathroom). Addressing a treatable cause of a problem behavior or a decline in function (for example, obtaining medical treatment for a bladder infection) can lead to a dramatic reduction in the unwanted behavior.

## General Suggestions

### Simplify the Environment

A busy, cluttered, and confusing environment can add to the anxiety and disorientation a memory-disordered person already feels because of his cognitive deficits. Behaviors such as pacing, fearfulness, restlessness, and unwillingness to cooperate may be triggered by a confusing environment. Communicating with your family member will be easier when distractions and sources of possible confusion are reduced. Without totally disrupting your life-style, look for ways to make the physical environment of the home and the impaired person's room free of unnecessary clutter and confusion.

Simple furnishings, good lighting, and as much space as possible to move around in will help to prevent or reduce some undesirable behaviors. Once things are reorganized to your satisfaction, avoid changing furniture arrangements and other physical features of the environment to the degree that you can. A calm, uncluttered environment "communicates" a sense of control and security to the person with dementia. This ideal kind of setting for the impaired individual is not always easy or even possible to achieve, but you can keep working on it.

## Make the Environment Safe and Secure

In addition to simplifying the environment, you will want to make your home as safe and secure for your family member as you can. Keep in mind that he will gradually lose the ability to understand your verbal admonitions to be careful, to turn off the stove, or to cool the hot water before getting in the tub. Your family member will, in time, no longer have the cognitive and communication abilities to appreciate what is dangerous to himself and to others.

If he is a smoker, fire danger is a real concern as judgment and memory abilities diminish. If your relative continues to smoke, you may want to discuss possible ways to encourage him to give up cigarettes with his physician or another member of the dementia care team. It may be easier than you think to get the person with dementia to smoke only when supervised.

## Check for Potential Safety Hazards

The best way to avoid mishaps is to check your home carefully for potential hazards, in much the same way you would if there were young children in the home. At some point in the disease progression, you'll need to secure all medicines and dangerous household chemicals in locked cabinets. You will need to lock up any power tools or personal weapons that may be interesting or attractive but dangerous to the impaired individual.

If wandering is a problem, place locks or latches either quite high or low on the outside doors to reduce the chance that the impaired individual will notice them. Examine your home for items that might cause your family member to trip and fall, or otherwise injure himself. In time, you may have to safety proof your kitchen by removing knobs from the stove, for example.

Other specific ideas for making the environment safe and secure for the person with dementia can be found in the references listed in Chapter 17. The goal is not only to assure the safety of someone who can no longer do that for himself, but also to avoid communication difficulties over safety hazards by dealing with the potentially dangerous items in a preventive manner.

## Utilize Effective Communication Strategies

Many of the verbal and nonverbal communication techniques described in Chapters 6 through 9 will serve the dual purposes of improving communication between you and the impaired person and also of preventing or reducing problematic behaviors. Uncooperative behaviors and catastrophic reactions will be less frequent when your family member understands what you want. Fearfulness, frustration, anxiety, and refusal to participate socially can be reduced by a calm manner, accepting tone of voice, and reassuring touch. Remember to talk to the impaired person directly, face-to-face, using touch and gesture as well as speech to communicate. These techniques should increase the likelihood of his cooperation.

Generous praise and appropriate rewarding of acceptable efforts should increase the frequency of such behaviors. Keeping verbal messages short, direct, and simple improves the impaired person's ability to understand and reduces his confusion. Review the effective communication strategies suggested in earlier chapters if you're having difficulty with some of your relative's behaviors. Communicating with him in a different way may be at least part of the answer.

## Look for Physical Reasons for Behavior Changes

Changes, especially sudden changes, in your relative's behavior may indicate a physical problem such as illness or infection. Since he may be unable to communicate discomfort or pain to you verbally, you need to be alert to other signs that he may need medical attention. Be especially alert for any nonverbal cues he gives you, such as grimacing or wincing when being helped to dress or to bathe. Use simple communication techniques suggested in earlier chapters to determine whether he can show you a particular area of discomfort, or indicate what is bothering him when he is given verbal choices. Ask him questions related to pain or discomfort so that he can respond with "yes" or "no."

# Managing Troublesome Behaviors in the Early Stages of Dementia

Some of the problem behaviors you may see in the person with mild dementia include irritability, anger and frustration, depression, and denial. Each of these behaviors can be related, at least in part, to the communication losses the individual is experiencing.

## Irritability

The sense that something is wrong with his memory, word-finding, and thinking abilities, and that he is losing control over his environment can cause the person with mild dementia to be irritable. Irritability may also be a sign of early personality changes more directly related to the dementing illness. Patient, supportive listening, realistic reassurance that you are there for him, and pointing out his strengths may go a long way in reducing irritability. In some ways, having a diagnosis, a *reason* to explain some of the changes he is experiencing can be re-assuring. The person with mild dementia needs to know that he is not going "crazy" and that he is valued and appreciated. A supportive peer group of similarly affected individuals may be helpful at this time.

## Anger and Frustration

The mildly impaired person may show anger and frustration at specific communication lapses, at his inability to express himself in a given situation. He may also become angry with you when you cannot interpret his sometimes jumbled verbal messages. Use some of the communication techniques you've learned to "hear him out" and to show him that you are trying to understand.

Keeping calm and not reacting to anger directed at you (no easy task!) can help. Try to determine whether this anger and frustration is associated with particular situations or times of day. Confusion in the environment and fatigue may be contributing.

Review the communication suggestions in Chapters 6 and 7, such as giving the impaired individual time to find the word he is looking for, reducing background noise, and diplomatically providing cues to get the conversation back on track. These ideas will hopefully reduce anger and frustration that is based on communication difficulty.

If he appears to be angry about something other than a communication problem, use your listening skills and question-asking abilities to try to determine the cause of the anger. Remember to phrase questions simply and to ask one question at a time. Appreciating that the anger is probably not really directed at you, but at his situation and diminishing abilities can help you accept your family member's outbursts and deal with them calmly.

## Depression

Depressed mood and feelings of discouragement and hopelessness can be seen in early-stage dementia. Lack of interest in activities and in people whose company he previously enjoyed, lack of interest in eating, and sleeping problems can be signs that your family member may be depressed because of his situation and the losses he is experiencing.

Obtain a medical evaluation of your family member's mood if you think that he may be depressed. It is possible that your loved one will function better despite his dementing illness if he is treated for depression. Depression is one of the treatable conditions accompanying Alzheimer's disease.

At the same time, supportive listening, allowing him to do as much for himself as he can, and frequent reassurance from you can help to improve his mood and his sense of self-worth.

# Denial

Early in the course of Alzheimer's disease, the impaired person may deny that anything is wrong with his memory or thinking abilities. He may become angry and upset if mistakes are pointed out to him. This denial can be the impaired person's way of coping with losses of which he is aware, or with a devastating prognosis. It does little good to argue with your relative if he shifts the blame for memory lapses to you or to other members of the family. In fact, a rule of thumb should be *don't* argue or get into a verbal tug-of-war with your impaired family member. Do what you can to distract him, or ignore the denial. In time, this will work itself out.

There are some situations, however, in which you cannot simply ignore his protests that he is as capable as ever. If, for example, he should continue to insist on driving the car when you and others consider him unsafe to be on the road, you will have to deal with it directly. You may need to take the car keys and hide them in a secure place. Consult with your relative's physician, psychologist, or social worker for other suggestions on dealing with driving issues. Other members of your Alzheimer's family support group may have ideas that worked for them. If driving privileges are relinquished, your loved one may need some special support and reassurance from you to deal with yet another significant loss.

## Managing Difficult Behaviors Associated with Moderate Dementia

In the middle or moderate phase of dementing illness, problematic behaviors may include wandering, restlessness, suspiciousness, hallucinations, catastrophic reactions, and changes in the person's wake-sleep patterns. As was true in the early or mild phase of the illness, management strategies should be aimed at *prevention* of problem behaviors to the extent possible. At this stage, it is important to recognize that the impaired person has little understanding of the impacts of his behavior on others and significantly impaired ability to learn and to adapt to his environment. His disturbing behaviors are rarely under his control at this stage. They are part of the disease process itself in some instances and result from environmental factors in other cases. Physical illnesses, such as infections, can trigger or exaggerate difficult behaviors.

In the middle stages of Alzheimer's disease, it is the caregiver who must change and adapt if disruptive behaviors are to be prevented or managed successfully when they do occur.

## Wandering

Wandering, or the impaired person's tendency to continue trying to leave his present environment, is commonly seen in the middle stages of dementing illness. It is still a somewhat poorly understood behavior and appears to be related to the disease process itself. Wandering may be the result of the person's disorientation and confusion in a new or strange environment, an attempt to "go home" to a familiar and secure place. With time, the impaired person will not even recognize familiar surroundings as "home" and may wander in search of a remembered home. The person with moderate dementia may also wander because he is bored or restless. Wandering can sometimes be an impaired person's way of "escaping" from an environment he perceives as threatening and unsafe.

### Managing Wandering Behavior

Strategies for managing wandering behavior include preventive measures such as securing the environment, especially access to the out-of-doors; providing time for walks and other gentle exercise; and making the environment as safe as possible to allow the impaired person some freedom and mobility. Staying with your family member for a while in a new or unfamiliar setting can be reassuring to him, and reduce his need to wander. Keeping him busy and occupied in suitable activities can lessen the frequency of wandering behavior. Distracting the wandering person when he seems determined to go can sometimes work. Inviting your family member to have a cup of tea or a glass of juice, to watch a television program, or listen to some favorite music can be effective in temporarily counteracting the need to wander.

For your peace of mind and your family member's safety, obtain a "medic-alert" identification bracelet (see Chapter 17, under Helpful Organizations and Agencies). Have the bracelet engraved with the words "memory impaired" or "memory disorder" and include the impaired person's name, address, and a telephone number where someone familiar with him can be reached. Make sure that your relative wears this important identification at all times. Another suggestion offered by many authors is to keep a current picture of your impaired relative on hand. This will be helpful to law enforcement agencies and others should he wander away from home and become lost.

## Restlessness

At times, the person with moderate dementia may fidget, pace back and forth, wring his hands, move the same objects around repeatedly, or continuously rummage through drawers. He may repeat the same question continuously, or fuss with his clothing. These restless behaviors may be seen even though the impaired individual doesn't try to leave the premises. In that respect, restless behaviors may be seen in people who are not "wanderers."

Restlessness can be an indication that your family member is anxious or afraid. It may be related to his inability to remember things for more than a brief time. He may be looking for something he believes he should be able to find, perhaps even an item from the distant past. Typically, the person with moderate dementia may not be able to communicate to you what is causing him to feel restless.

### Early Warning Signs

You will need to learn to recognize the "early warning signs" of restlessness to prevent the situation from triggering a *catastrophic reaction* (described later in this chapter). These early signals that the person is becoming restless occur before any obvious movement, such as pacing. They include the following: (1) Your relative stops making eye contact with you; (2) you can't engage him socially, or in conversation. If you see these signs, you should drop what you are doing immediately and make a change in the activity, or suggest a distraction that you know the person enjoys (a treat, a walk, some music perhaps). You have only a *short window of opportunity* to prevent a restless episode if you see these early warning signs.

### Examine the Environment

Look first for possible reasons within the environment for the person's restless behavior. Is a confusing environment or a large group of people making him feeling anxious and fearful? Does his behavior give you any clue as to what he might be searching for? Does your relative become restless only in certain places?

### Is There a Pattern to the Restless Behavior?

Do you see any pattern to your family member's restlessness? For example, does it occur at a certain time each day, or with particular people? Can you identify the "early warning signs"?

### Managing Restless Behavior

If anxiety and concern are causing the restless behavior, reassuring your relative in a calm and positive way that he is safe and that you are there to help him may be of benefit. Use the communication strategies described in this book to see if you can determine a reason for the behavior. It does little good to tell the memory-impaired person to stop the repetitive behavior, or to reprimand him for something that is not under his control. In fact, such negative communication may cause the individual to be more upset and could provoke a catastrophic reaction. A more effective technique would be to engage your family member in a pleasant activity. Distracting him may reduce the restless behavior. Responding to the early warning signs promptly is the best preventive approach.

## Suspiciousness

Suspiciousness is seen in some people with moderately severe dementia. The affected individual may believe that "Somebody is stealing from me" because he cannot remember where he has put things, or that he gave a particular item away some time ago. Some writers speculate that referring to things being "stolen" may be the impaired person's way of expressing the many losses he has experienced because of the disease. His memory, communication abilities, and other important functions are being "stolen" from him.

### Coping with Suspicious Behavior

How do you deal with accusations directed at you or other members of the family? It can hurt deeply when your family member says that you have taken all of his money when you're working day and night to provide good care for him. One thing to keep in mind is that the *feeling* being expressed by your impaired family member may be accurate. He knows that he once had something. Now he cannot find the item, therefore it must have been stolen, since he has no other explanation. He is feeling a loss. For example, when the impaired individual who has had his driving privileges taken away says that "Somebody stole my car," he may be expressing the loss he feels because he can no longer drive.

In responding to the suspicious person with dementia, try to get beyond the words themselves and to the feeling he might be attempting to express. Don't argue with him that no one has stolen his car, that it was sold several months ago with his permission. Instead, empathize with what he is expressing by saying, for example, "It must be hard not to be driving yourself places any more. We're happy to see that you get wherever you need to go."

## Hallucinations

Some people with moderate dementia may imagine that they see, hear, or smell people or things that are not there.

They can also misinterpret environmental stimuli such as wall fixtures or voices coming over the radio. These are called *hallucinations*, and they can be very frightening to the person who experiences them.

If your family member has hallucinations, you will want to avoid directly confronting him or arguing with him that "nothing is there, you're just imagining it." Keep in mind that the hallucination is very real to the person experiencing it. Instead of confrontation, you can sometimes effectively call your relative back to the "here and now" by saying his name, perhaps accompanying it with a gentle touch.

If the hallucination is visibly upsetting to the person, you may have to respond with a reality-oriented statement. For example, if the impaired individual is saying "This person is trying to kill me with a knife!" you should respond with something like, "There is no one here with a knife. I'm here and I love you. You're safe here." If hallucinations continue to upset your family member, you should discuss the problem with his physician or with the dementia team. A medication prescribed by a professional who knows your relative can be helpful in these circumstances.

## Catastrophic Reactions

There may be times when your relative overreacts to a suggestion or request, seemingly out of proportion to what was just said to him or to what was going on at the moment. You may have been trying to convince him that it was time for a bath when the anger outburst occurred.

These uncontrolled, unexpected outbursts are known as *catastrophic reactions*. The cognitively impaired person's behavior suggests that a catastrophe has occurred when that is not the case. The person with moderate dementia has little control over or insight into these reactions. He may be striking out because of the loss of control he feels in an increasingly confusing environment.

### Managing Catastrophic Reactions

The goal in managing difficult behaviors is to *prevent* catastrophic reactions from occurring, through the use of effective communication strategies and structuring of the environment of the impaired person. Dealing with troublesome behaviors in a positive way before they become full-blown outbursts should be an achievable goal in most situations. There may be those times, however, when your best efforts cannot prevent a catastrophic reaction.

People in the impaired individual's environment need to act calmly and purposefully when a catastrophic reaction occurs, or when they see that the person is becoming highly agitated. Some writers have suggested that the caregiver needs to remember "The Five Rs": *Remain calm.* You don't want to confront the person or argue with him. *Respond* to what you sense the person is feeling, if you can determine what might be the emotion underlying the reaction. *Reassure* the person that he is in a safe place, and that things are all right. *Remove* yourself from the situation if necessary, especially if you are in danger of being injured by the upset individual. *Return* later, when the person has calmed down again.

## Incontinence

Incontinence, the loss of bladder and bowel control, is not usually seen until the later stages of dementing illness. There are sometimes medical or physical reasons for the incontinence, especially if it is experienced by someone with mild dementia. In such a situation, a medical evaluation to determine possible reasons for the loss of control needs to be completed. In the person with moderate dementia, there may be communication-related or environmentally related reasons for incontinence. Perhaps the impaired person is unable to express his need to use the bathroom. Perhaps he is confused and cannot find the toilet, especially at night.

### Managing Incontinence

Incontinence may be successfully dealt with for a time by asking the memory-impaired person regularly (every couple of hours) if he needs to use the toilet. A sign on the bathroom door and a night light can be helpful in reducing or eliminating some incontinence problems, as can having a urinal or commode handy in the affected individual's bedroom at night. Eliminating liquids a few hours before bedtime will cut down on nighttime incontinence.

Incontinence is a complex problem, with many possible causes and different management strategies for individuals' specific needs. If incontinence is a problem for your relative, seek the advice of his physician or the dementia team. They're there to help you, and they have expert advice to share. You may want to refer to another book in this series, *Coping with Bowel and Bladder Problems*, by Barbara King and Judy Harke for more information on how to deal with incontinence issues.

## Disturbance of Sleep-Wake Cycles

It is not uncommon for the person in the middle stages of dementing illness to experience "sundowning," that is, a disturbance in the normal body cycles of wakefulness and sleeping. The individual who is displaying sundowning tends to be awake at night, even up and wandering about, and sleepy during the day. Dementia has disturbed those biological signals in the brain that tell us whether it is night or day. Furthermore, the individual may no longer be able to process the environmental cues we use to recognize that it's time to go to bed, or that we've gotten up too early. This can wreak havoc on the caregiver who is not able to get proper rest because her relative is up and trying to put his clothes on in the middle of the night.

### Strategies for Dealing with Sleep-Wakefulness Problems

There are a few "communication strategies" in dealing with this disturbance of the wake-sleep cycle that might work for you.

1. Make sure that your relative puts pajamas on (if he is used to sleeping in pajamas) as a "cue" that it is bedtime.
2. Put his daytime clothes out of sight at night, so that they are not readily available to him.

3. During the day, even if your relative enjoys a nap, don't put him to bed to nap if sundowning is a problem. That may confuse him, and he may think it is nighttime because of the environmental cue of going to his bed.

4. Instead, have him rest or nap in a lounge chair, or on the sofa during the day.

5. Plan some activities, including exercise, to keep your family member stimulated so that he will be tired at night.

6. Discuss the situation with the physician who is caring for your relative or with the dementia team if you find that the impaired person is turning night into day and vice versa.

# Managing Problem Behaviors in Dementia's Late Stages

By the time dementing illness has reached the severe and final stages, many of the problem behaviors that were encountered earlier in the illness, such as wandering, suspiciousness, and agitation are no longer evident. The person is less mobile, perhaps bedbound, and his physical care becomes a major focus. Nevertheless there are some new problems to confront as your family member becomes more severely impaired. Eating and swallowing problems, for example, will present challenges in dementia's final stages.

## Eating/Swallowing Problems

Gradually, the person with dementing illness will lose the ability to associate food with its purpose. He may forget that he is supposed to swallow. He may, in the final stages of dementia, lose all memory of the sequences of motor movements involved in swallowing, or lose the physical ability to swallow itself.

This can be very upsetting to you as the caregiver, even though you may understand the reasons for these eating difficulties. We tend to view providing nourishment as a sign of love and caring. Food has great symbolic value in our culture as in most others. You may feel that providing food and liquid for your loved one is one of the few ways in which you still "communicate." Then again, you've likely been counseled throughout his illness that good nutrition is important to your family member. You may be feeling guilty if you observe that your loved one is not eating or drinking enough.

Here are a few general suggestions for managing feeding and swallowing difficulties in the severe stages of dementia.

### Choose Foods That are Easier to Swallow

If your family member is no longer able to chew foods easily, you may want to prepare blenderized or pureed foods for him. These can be made flavorful. You can puree many of his favorite foods for easier swallowing. Liquids such as milkshakes or nutritional supplements may be both easier to swallow and provide extra calories if that is a concern. A registered dietitian can help you select nourishing, nutritionally balanced, and appropriate liquid diet supplements. Dietitians are often available to assist you as members of dementia care teams, or through a home health agency.

### Verbal Cuing May Be Necessary

You may observe that your family member tends to keep food presented to him in his mouth, perhaps seeming to chew on it, but not remembering to swallow. For those individuals who have forgotten that they need to swallow food and liquids, a verbal prompt to swallow can cue them to complete the swallowing sequence. When feeding someone who seems to need these verbal cues it's important to make sure that the previous bite of food has been swallowed before presenting another.

### Eliminate or Reduce Distractions

In the later stages of dementing illness, environmental distractions such as noise, other activity going on in the eating area, or people talking can catch the attention of the impaired person when you are trying to get him to eat. This can cause him to forget to swallow, or you may see a delayed swallow. As much as possible, reduce mealtime noise and confusion so that your family member can attend to the task of eating. Find a quiet spot for meal times, and make sure that the television and radio are turned off, at a minimum.

### Present Small Amounts of Food at a Time

A full plate of food can seem overwhelming to the person with severe cognitive problems and a diminished appetite. Your relative might respond better and improve his eating if you present just one food item at a time. You might also try saving some of the items (such as pudding or custard for dessert) for a later snack. A person with severe dementia may do better with several small meals and snacks a day rather than three large or average-size meals. Remember also that in the later stages of Alzheimer's disease, an individual's appetite may be reduced.

### Consider Talking with a Dietician

The person with severe dementia may begin to lose weight as part of the progressive process of the disease. At the same time, eating and swallowing may become difficult for him. He may begin refusing nourishment as well. If you are concerned about your family member's weight loss, or think that he is not getting enough fluids, talk to his physician about this. A clinical dietitian can offer specific suggestions to increase calories if that is recommended. If your family member has been followed by a dementia team, you may already have consulted regularly with a dietitian. If not, you may want to make an appointment at this time to discuss your family member's food and fluid needs.

### Position the Person for Safety

When swallowing becomes difficult for the impaired person, you will want to pay special attention to how he is positioned when taking food or liquids by mouth. Careful positioning will reduce the chances that anything he eats or drinks gets into his windpipe or lungs. If your family member is able to sit up and is able to walk some, even with assistance, have him sit at a table for meals. If this is no longer possible and you must feed him in bed, be sure that he is sitting as upright in bed as possible.

### Present Food and Liquid When the Person is Alert and Awake

The chances of your family member getting food or liquid into his windpipe and lungs (called *aspiration*) may be increased if he is drowsy and not alert. Present food and liquids when your relative is most alert and awake.

### Formal Swallowing Evaluations

It has already been suggested that you might want to talk with a dietitian if you are concerned about your family member's nutrition and whether he is getting adequate fluids. Other members of the health care team can be helpful to you as well.

Your relative may be evaluated by a *speech-language pathologist*, a professional who is qualified by education and training to provide assistance related to communication concerns as well as certain types of swallowing problems. This individual will be able to evaluate whether the muscles used to prepare food for swallowing and to begin the act of swallowing are functioning properly. The speech-language pathologist may recommend a special x-ray study, called a *barium swallow*, to determine whether your family member is aspirating when he eats or drinks. This study would be performed by a medical specialist, a *radiologist*. After the swallowing evaluation is complete, the speech-language pathologist will offer you suggestions to lessen the risk of aspiration when your family member eats and drinks.

### When Swallowing Problems Become Severe

If eating problems become severe, caregivers are often faced with the difficult decision of whether to consider some other means of nutrition for their loved one, such as a feeding tube. Deciding whether to have a feeding tube placed in someone with severe dementia is never an easy decision to make. You need to discuss your feelings about the issue of tube feeding for your relative with the physician or the dementia team, preferably before you need to make a decision when you are stressed. Perhaps your relative has expressed his preferences regarding feeding issues when he was still cognitively able to do so. He may have expressed them to you verbally or in a written document. You'll want to share this information with the health care team as well. Remember that the team is there to assist you in weighing these difficult choices.

# A Final Word About Problem Behaviors

This chapter has touched on some of the problem behaviors you may or may not encounter in caring for your family member. Your relative's behaviors may be similar to those described here or present unique challenges of their own. The resources listed in Chapter 17 contain many more ideas and suggestions for managing the difficult behaviors that can be part of Alzheimer's disease. Remember that good communication skills can be a big help in reducing the occurrence of some problem behaviors. For others, you should seek guidance from a knowledgeable physician or from other members of the dementia care team. It's important that you realize you're not alone in coping with these behavioral challenges.

# Chapter 16

# Some Concluding Thoughts

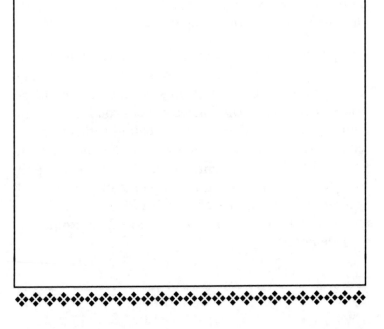

The theme of this book has been communication in its broadest sense. As the caregiver of someone with dementia, you have faced communication challenges from the moment that the dementing illness was diagnosed, and perhaps before then. You may have had to work long and hard to convince your family member that a medical evaluation should be sought. You may have struggled to ask the right questions of the physician and other health care providers who first gave you and your loved one the news that a progressive dementia — Alzheimer's disease — was the likely cause of the changes he was experiencing. Most probably you have also had to communicate with other family members and close friends about the illness, some of whom may have had a difficult time accepting the diagnosis of dementia. You have likely had to communicate your needs for assistance to any number of agency personnel. And you have had to learn to modify and adapt your communication approaches to match your family member's changing abilities and insights.

The positive message that this book has attempted to convey is that in the face of a devastating illness characterized by many bleak moments, positive communication strategies *can help*. They can help you feel more in control and more confident in dealing with the challenges you face. They can help you see the humanity in your affected family member, as you learn different ways to communicate with him. Hopefully, successful communication approaches will reduce some of the stress that inevitably is part of caring for someone with dementia.

While there is no cure at present for Alzheimer's disease, and no way to restore lost communication abilities for the affected person, communication challenges *can* be effectively managed, to the benefit of both you and your family member.

This book has not touched on all of the communication issues that come up in the course of a dementing illness. Sooner or later, for example, you may be faced with the difficult decision of whether to place your family member in a nursing home or another type of care facility. Most people in the severe and final stages of dementing illness require more care than families can provide. If and when you are faced with this decision, you will be dealing with new communication issues — letting your family member know of your decision, asking the right questions of nursing home personnel, and communicating with facility staff about your loved one so that they will know something about the person he was. Several of the references in Chapter 17 offer suggestions for coping with the issue of nursing home placement. Other excellent resources are the Alzheimer's Association and their local chapters and the American Association of Retired Persons.

Finally, the one important person you need to keep communicating with is yourself. You must let yourself know what *your* needs are throughout this process of caregiving. You are not being selfish in considering your physical, emotional, and psychological needs, for it is the only way you can continue to provide the care your loved one requires. Keep in touch with yourself — your feelings, your accomplishments, your stresses, your need for relaxation and small pleasures. You deserve it — you're doing a splendid job!

# Chapter 17

# Useful Resources

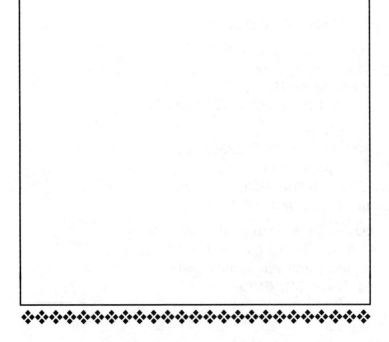

In this chapter, you will find additional sources of information and assistance. First, there is a listing of agencies and organizations that can provide specific kinds of help. This is followed by a selected list of reading materials and videotapes that will give you more information on areas of specific concern, such as dealing with legal matters, managing problem behaviors, or choosing a good nursing home. Some of the books listed are personal accounts of how individuals and families have met the challenges of Alzheimer's disease. Others have been written especially for children and adolescents. It is hoped that, as you utilize some of these resources, you will become more aware that you and your family are not coping with this disease alone.

# Helpful Organizations and Agencies

### National Organizations

Administration on Aging
330 Independence Avenue
Washington, DC 20201
General Information: (202) 245-0011

Alzheimer's Association, Inc.
70 East Lake Street, Suite 600
Chicago, IL 60601
(312) 853-3060; (800) 621-0379;
in Illinois, (800) 572-6037

American Affiliation of Visiting Nurse
  Associations and Services
21 Maryland Plaza, Suite 300
St. Louis, MO 63108

American Association of Homes for the Aging
1129 20th Street NW, Suite 400
Washington, DC 20036
(202) 296-5960

American Association of Retired Persons
1909 K Street NW
Washington, DC 20049
(202) 872-4700

American Federation of Home Health Agencies
429 N Street SW, Suite S-605
Washington, DC 20024

American Geriatrics Society
770 Lexington Avenue, Suite 400
New York, NY 10021
(212) 308-1414

American Health Care Association
1200 15th Street NW
Washington, DC 20005
(202) 833-2050

American Society on Aging
833 Market Street, Suite 516
San Francisco, CA 94103
(415) 543-2617

American Speech-Language-Hearing
   Association (ASHA)
10801 Rockville Pike
Rockville, MD 20852
(301) 897-5700

Asociacion Nacional pro Persones Mayores
(National Association for Hispanic Elderly)
2727 West 6th Street, Room 270
Los Angeles, CA 90057
(213) 487-1922

The Gerontological Society of America
1411 K Street NW, Suite 300
Washington, DC 20005
(202) 393-1411

Gray Panthers
311 S. Juniper Street, Suite 601
Philadelphia, PA 19107
(215) 545-6555

Health Care Financing Administration
200 Independence Avenue SW
Washington, DC 20201
(202) 245-6726

Medic-Alert Foundation International
1000 North Palm Street
Turlock, CA 95380

National Association of Area Agencies on Aging
600 Maryland Avenue SW
West Wing, Suite 208
Washington, DC 20024
(202) 484-7520

National Association of State Units on Aging
600 Maryland Avenue SW
West Wing, Suite 208
Washington, DC 20024
(202) 484-7182

National Caucus and Center on Black Aged
1424 K Street NW, Suite 500
Washington, DC 20005
(202) 637-0657

National Council of Senior Citizens
1331 F Street
Washington, DC 20004
(919) 347-8800

National Council on Black Aging
Box 8813
Durham, NC 27707
(919) 489-2563

National Indian Council on Aging
P.O. Box 2088
Albuquerque, NM 87103
(505) 242-9500

National Institute on Aging
Public Information Office
Building 31, Room 5C 35
9000 Rockville Pike
Bethesda, MD 20892
(301) 496-1752

National Institution on Adult Day Care
600 Maryland Avenue SW
West Wing, Suite 100
Washington, DC 20024

National Pacific/Asian Resource Center on Aging
811 First Avenue
Colman Building, Suite 212

Seattle, WA 98112
(206) 622-5124

National Senior Citizens Law Center
2025 M Street NW, Suite 400
Washington, DC 20036

## Useful Hotlines

*Alcohol Abuse Hotline* 1-800-ALCOHOL. Operates 24 hours a day, 7 days a week. Provides counseling for caregivers or family members with dementia who have alcohol problems.

*Grief Hotline:* (312) 990-0010. An organization called the Compassionate Friends will provide referrals for caregivers who have recently lost a loved one. Operates 9 a.m. to 3 p.m. CST, Monday through Friday.

*Home Care Hotline:* (202) 547-7424. The National Association for Home Care provides referrals concerning local medical home care organizations. Operates 9 a.m. to 6 p.m. EST, Monday through Friday.

*Pain Control Hotline:* (703) 368-7357. Operates 24 hours a day, 7 days a week. Answers all questions pertaining to pain control. (They will call back collect if no one answers and you leave a message on their answering machine.)

*Suicide Hotline:* (213) 381-5111. Operates 24 hours a day, 7 days a week. Provides immediate telephone counseling for people who are contemplating suicide or for people with family members at high suicide risk. Can refer callers to suicide prevention clinics.

*Surgical Second Opinion Hotline:* (800) 638-6833. A government-sponsored service providing information on where to get a second opinion on proposed surgical operations. Operates 8 a.m. to midnight, 7 days a week.

## Suggested Local Sources of Help

Local chapter of the *Alzheimer's Association*

*Local Family Service Agencies* (Check in the telephone directory under Social Service Agencies or Social Service Organizations)

*Counseling Services.* Check with:
Hospital Social Work Departments
Mental Health Clinics
Churches and Synagogues
Senior Citizen Centers
Senior Housing
Long-term Care Facilities

# General Books

Aronson, M. K. (Ed.). Alzheimer's Disease and Related Disorders Association. (1988). *Alzheimer's disease: What it is; how to cope with it; future directions.* New York: Charles Scribner's Sons. Written for the general reader, this book contains chapters by several prominent people in the field of dementia. Provides a comprehensive overview of dementing disorders, management and coping strategies.

Blevins, E. L., Darnell, L. J., & Bonebrake, C. C. (1987). *The nursing home and you: Partners in caring for a rela-*

*tive with Alzheimer's disease.* Washington, DC: American Association of Homes for the Aging. Helpful suggestions for those whose relative with dementia is now in a nursing home, or for whom nursing home placement is being considered.

Carroll, D. L. (1989). *When your loved one has Alzheimer's disease. A caregiver's guide.* New York: Harper and Row. Based on methods developed at the Brookdale Center on Aging. Practical suggestions for dealing with some of the common problems faced by caregivers of people with dementia.

Cohen, D., & Eisdorfer, C. (1986). *The loss of self.* New York: W. W. Norton. An excellent and sensitive book that focuses on the humanity of the person afflicted with Alzheimer's disease. Covers most aspects of coping with Alzheimer's disease.

Dippel, R. L., & Hutton, J. T. (Eds.). (1988). *Caring for the Alzheimer patient: A practical guide* (2nd ed.). Buffalo, NY: Prometheus Books. A general book covering many topics of concern to families and friends of dementia victims. Multiple authors have addressed the different topics.

Gruetzner, H. (1988). *Alzheimer's: A caregiver's guide and sourcebook.* New York: John Wiley & Sons. An overview and resource book that contains background information on Alzheimer's disease (including definitions, causes, research). Two chapters deal with management issues of concern to caregivers.

Gwyther, L. P. (1985). *Care of Alzheimer's patients: A manual for nursing home staff.* Washington, DC: American Health Care Association; Chicago, IL: Alzheimer's Disease and Related Disorders Association, Inc. (Alzheimer's Association). Although written for nursing home staff, this manual also contains helpful information for family and other informal caregivers.

Heston, L., & White, J. (1983). *Dementia: A practical guide to Alzheimer's disease and related illnesses.* New York: W. H. Freeman & Co. This text provides an overview of the dementing illnesses, including Alzheimer's disease. The authors describe the signs and symptoms of dementia and discuss diseases associated with various dementing conditions. Causes of dementia, treatment issues, and suggestions for dealing with practical concerns are included.

Horne, J. (1989). *The nursing home handbook.* Washington, DC: American Association of Retired Persons. Glenview, IL: Scott, Foresman and Co. Contains practical advice and information to assist families in making the difficult decisions involved in placing a loved one in a nursing home. Included are a comprehensive check list with which to evaluate facilities before a placement decision is made and suggestions for working with nursing home staff.

Kalicki, A. C. (Ed.). (1987). *Confronting Alzheimer's disease.* Washington, DC: National Health. An overview of Alzheimer's disease. Written for nursing home administrators as well as for family members. Not overly technical.

Kindig, M., & Carnes, M. (in press). *Coping with Alzheimer's disease and other dementing illnesses.* San Diego, CA: Singular Publishing Group.

Mace, N., & Rabins, P. (1991). *The 36-hour day: A family guide to caring for persons with Alzheimer's disease, related dementing illnesses, and memory loss in later life* (Rev. ed.). Baltimore, MD: Johns Hopkins University Press. This classic text has been recently revised. Probably the most frequently recommended book on Alzheimer's disease for families.

Miner, G. D., Winters-Miner, L. A., Blass, J. P., Richter, R. W., & Valentine, J. L. (1989). *Caring for Alzheimer's patients. A guide for family and healthcare providers.* New York: Plenum Press. Focus is on the familial type of Alzheimer's disease, but contains useful information on dealing with the broader issues of dementia.

Oliver, R., & Bock, F. A. (1987). *Coping with Alzheimer's: A caregiver's emotional survival guide.* New York: Dodd, Mead. This book focuses on the myriad of emotions and feelings experienced over the course of caring for someone with a dementing illness and on suggestions for dealing with these feelings.

Ostuni, E., & Santo Pietro, M. J. (1986). *Getting through: Communicating when someone you care for has Alzheimer's disease.* Princeton Junction, NJ: The Speech Bin. Useful, practical suggestions focusing on communication issues.

Powell, L. S., & Courtice, K. (1983). *Alzheimer's disease. A guide for families.* Reading, MA: Addison-Wesley. Overview of caregiving issues and concerns.

Robinson, A., Spencer, B., & White, L. (1989). *Understanding difficult behaviors.* Geriatric Education Center of Michigan, Series on Alzheimer's disease and related illnesses. Ypsilanti, MI: Eastern Michigan University. Out-lines specific difficult behaviors commonly seen in individuals with Alzheimer's disease and strategies for coping with them.

Ronch, J. L. (1989). *Alzheimer's disease. A practical guide for those who help others.* New York: Continuum. Written primarily for health care professionals who counsel families dealing with dementing illness.

Safford, F. (1989). *Caring for the mentally impaired elderly: A family guide.* New York: Henry Holt. Contains several chapters that explain the terminology, symptoms, and causes of mental impairment in the elderly. There are useful suggestions regarding communicating with health care professionals and dealing with upsetting problems that arise in providing day-to-day care.

Sheridan, C. (1987). *Failure-free activities for the Alzheimer's patient: A guidebook for caregivers.* Oakland, CA: Cottage Books. Suggestions of activities to stimulate the Alzheimer's patient.

Stokes, G., & Goudie, F. (1990). *Working with dementia.* Bicester, UK: Winslow Press. Written primarily for people working in long-term care settings, but contains information helpful to family members of people with dementia as well. A hopeful book focusing on "relearning and rehabilitation" strategies that allow the individual with dementia to function optimally within the limitations caused by the disease.

Zgola, J. M. (1987). *Doing things: A guide to programming activities for persons with Alzheimer's disease.* Baltimore, MD: Johns Hopkins University Press. This is a guide for professionals and volunteers involved in adult day care programs, as well as for home caregivers. Contains a wealth of suggestions for planning simple, pleasurable, success-oriented activities for people with dementia.

## Books for Children

Delton, J., Tucker, D., & Robinson, C. (1986). *My grandma's in a nursing home.* Niles, IL: Albert Whitman and Co.

Guthrie, D. (1986). *Grandpa doesn't know it's me.* New York: Human Sciences Press.

Kibbey, M. (1988). *My granny.* Minneapolis, MN: Carolrhoda Books.

Rappaport, D. (1982). *But she's still my grandma!* New York: Human Sciences Press.

Sanford, D., & Evans, G. (1989). *Maria's grandma gets mixed up.* Portland, OR: Multnomah Press.

## Books for Teenagers

Frank, J. (1985). *The silent epidemic.* Minneapolis, MN: Lerner Publications Co.

Young, A. E. (1986). *What's wrong with daddy?* Worthington, OH: Willowisp Press.

## Personal Accounts (Caregivers and Dementia Victims)

Atkins, M. (1985). *Also my journey.* Wilton, CT: Morehouse Publishing.

Ball, A. J. (1986). *Caring for an aging parent: Have I done all I can?* Buffalo, NY: Prometheus Books.

Bauer, C. (1987). *When I grow too old to dream: A journal on Alzheimer's disease.* New York: Vantage Press.

Brown, D. S. (1984). *Handle with care: A question of Alzheimer's.* Buffalo, NY: Prometheus Books. A daughter's account of her experiences in caring for her mother, a dementia victim.

Bryan, J. (Ed.). (1987). *Love is ageless: Stories about Alzheimer's disease.* Oakland, CA: Serala Press. A collection of essays and vignettes reflecting the personal experiences with dementia of the different authors.

Davis, R. (1989). *My journey into Alzheimer's disease.* Wheaton, IL: Tyndale House Publishers. The author was a prominent and successful clergyman when he received the diagnosis of probable Alzheimer's disease. Written from a Christian faith perspective.

Doernberg, M. (1989). *Stolen mind: The slow disappearance of Ray Doernberg.* Chapel Hill, NC: Algonquin. A wife relates the story of her husband's dementing illness.

Holland, G. (1985). *For Sasha with love: An Alzheimer's crusade.* New York: Dembner Books.

Honel, R.W. (1988). *Journey with grandpa: Our family's struggle with Alzheimer's disease.* Baltimore, MD: Johns Hopkins University Press. The story is told by a daughter-in-law. This family story includes children growing up in the home of someone with Alzheimer's disease.

Roach, M. (1985). *Another name for madness.* Boston: Houghton-Mifflin. A daughter's account of the progression of her mother's Alzheimer's disease and its impacts on the family.

Seymour, C. (1983). *Precipice. Learning to live with Alzheimer's disease.* New York: Vantage Press. A spouse's personal account of her husband's Alzheimer's disease and their life together after his diagnosis. Written from a Christian faith perspective.

## Videotapes

*Alzheimer's disease – stolen tomorrows.* 1986. Van Nuys, CA: AIMS Media. 26 minutes. Family members share thoughts and experiences as they learn to cope with the symptoms of Alzheimer's disease. The stages of the disease are described and ways of dealing with the emotional and financial stresses that accompany the diagnosis are discussed.

Medical Media Production Service, Veterans Administration Medical Center, Northport, NY. *Alzheimer's disease: Managing the later stages in the home.* 1989. Washington, DC: Department of Veterans Affairs. 15 minutes. Provides caregivers with information to help them effectively manage the later stages of Alzheimer's disease in the home environment. The videotape addresses specific problems such as the Alzheimer's disease victim's personal safety, emotional well-being, personal comfort, feeding difficulties, and incontinence.

The Ramsey Foundation. *Dealing with Alzheimer's disease: A common-sense approach to communication.* 1990. Chicago, IL: Terra Nova Films, Inc. 21 minutes. The tape discusses and demonstrates a variety of successful communication techniques for caregivers of people with dementia.

*Designing the environment for persons with dementia.* 1987. Chicago, IL: Terra Nova Films, Inc. 20 minutes. Especially geared toward long-term care settings, but some of the interventions could be applied in the home as well.

*Wesley Hall: A special life.* 1987. Chicago, IL: Terra Nova Films, Inc. 28 minutes. Describes the development and philosophy of a special unit for people with dementia within a long-term care facility.

# Appendix

# A Glossary of Dementia-Related Terms

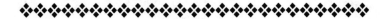

**ACTIVITIES OF DAILY LIVING (ADLs)** Functions of everyday life, including bathing, eating, dressing, grooming, going to the bathroom, and walking or getting about in other ways.

**AMBULATORY** Term used to describe an individual who is able to walk and move about, possibly with the aid of a device such as a cane or a walker. May include people who are able to get around (ambulate) in a wheelchair independently.

**ALZHEIMER'S DISEASE** A progressive, irreversible brain disorder that is gradual in onset and is characterized by deterioration of memory, communication skills, thinking abilities, personality, and behavior. There is at present no known cause and no known cure for the disease. It is the most common form of dementia, and it affects an estimated 2 to 4 million Americans.

**ANOMIA** Difficulty coming up with specific words because of damage or injury to the brain.

**APHASIA** Loss or decrease in the ability to use and to understand words or other language symbols (such as gestures) due to brain damage.

**APRAXIA** Difficulty in planning and carrying out a sequence of motor movements due to brain damage. In Alzheimer's disease, apraxia may result in problems with dressing, ambulation, or eating, for example.

**CATASTROPHIC REACTION** A term used to describe overreactions to situations that overwhelm the limited capacities of the person with brain disease. These overreactions may take the form of crying, anger, refusal to cooperate, or physically aggressive behavior.

**COMPETENCY** A legal term that refers to the power to manage one's own personal, financial, and/or legal affairs.

**COMPUTERIZED TOMOGRAPHY (CT) SCAN OF THE BRAIN** A special x-ray study of the brain that can provide information about the size and relationship of brain structures to one another. It can also detect the presence of certain brain diseases or damage (strokes, brain tumors, blood clots, or abnormal amounts of fluid). A diagnosis of Alzheimer's disease would not be made on the basis of a CT scan alone.

**CONSERVATOR** A person appointed by the court to manage the assets of a person who is considered legally incompetent (see **INCOMPETENCY**).

**DEMENTIA OF THE ALZHEIMER'S TYPE (DAT)** see **ALZHEIMER'S DISEASE.**

**DEHYDRATION** A condition in which the body has inadequate amounts of fluid (water). Signs of dehydration include dry skin, worsening mental functioning, and light output during urination. This can be a problem in advanced Alzheimer's disease, if fluid intake is poor or the person has trouble swallowing. Beverages that contain caffeine (coffee and tea) reduce body fluids because they are diuretics.

**DELUSION** A false or inaccurate personal belief that is firmly sustained despite all evidence to the contrary.

**DEMENTIA** Decline in memory, judgment, and higher intellectual functions from a person's previous level of functioning. Dementia may be caused by a number of diseases, the most common of which is Alzheimer's disease (AD).

**DIURETICS** Medications or other substances that cause the body to get rid of fluids by increasing urination.

**DURABLE POWER OF ATTORNEY** A written, legal document that lets an individual designate another person to act on his behalf. A Durable Power of Attorney can be broad, giving power to manage and control all aspects of a person's life, or it can be limited to specific assets or activities, such as making health care decisions.

**GERIATRICIAN** A physician who is a specialist in treating age-related diseases and illnesses of older people.

**GERIATRICS** A branch of medicine that specializes in age-related diseases and illnesses in the elderly.

**GERONTOLOGY** The study of all aspects of adult development and aging and their consequences, including social and psychological factors.

**GUARDIAN (CONSERVATOR OF PERSON)** A court-appointed person who is designated to assume responsibility for the physical care and well-being of an individual whom the court finds no longer capable of caring for his personal needs.

**HALLUCINATION** A strongly experienced false perception of objects or persons seen or voices heard that is not apparent to anyone else.

**HOME CARE** A variety of services provided in the home, ranging from nursing care, paid companionship for the person with dementia, and therapies to assistance with homemaking chores and personal care (bathing, dressing). Usually arranged through a Home Health Agency or Home Care Agency, for a fee.

**INCOMPETENCY** A court-determined designation that an individual is not capable of managing his assets or caring for himself.

**INCONTINENCE** Loss of bowel and/or bladder control.

**LIVING WILL** A general term for a written document in which a person indicates how health care decisions are to be made if he is incapacitated and unable to make such decisions for himself.

**MEDICAID** A joint federal and state medical benefits program for the elderly and disabled whose incomes fall below a certain level. Eligibility requirements and reimbursement levels vary from state to state.

**MEDICARE** A federal health insurance program primarily designed to cover hospital care for people age 65 and over, regardless of income. Some short-term nursing home and home health care costs may be partially covered.

**MULTI-INFARCT DEMENTIA (MID)** Dementia caused by a loss of brain tissue resulting from a series of small, often imperceptible strokes.

**NEURITIC PLAQUES** One of the brain changes associated with Alzheimer's disease. Plaques are degenerating bits of nerve cells surrounding a core of fibrous material called amyloid. They are found outside nerve cells. Usually seen on autopsy at death. Plaques are seen in the brains of older, nondemented people as well, but in much fewer numbers.

**NEUROFIBRILLARY TANGLES** One of the specific brain changes associated with Alzheimer's disease and usually seen at autopsy. Tangles are pairs of fine nerve fibers twisted around each other and lying in the cell bodies of neurons. They are sometimes found in normal, aged human brains, but in smaller numbers.

**NEUROLOGIST** A physician who specializes in the diagnosis and treatment of diseases of the brain and nervous system.

**NEUROPSYCHOLOGIST** An individual who holds a graduate degree in psychology (Ph.D.) and who is trained to evaluate the relationship between brain function and behavior. Neuropsychologists evaluate learning, memory, judgment, and other cognitive functions in people who have or are suspected of having brain damage or brain disease.

**NEUROTRANSMITTERS** Chemicals released by the brain to communicate with other nerve cells. Acetylcholine and dopamine are two neurotransmitters.

**PARANOIA** A suspicion of others that is not based in reality.

**PARAPHASIA** Substitution of another word for the word actually meant. The substitution may be a word similar in meaning (sister for aunt) or similar in sound. At times, the substitution may be a "nonsense" word.

**PSEUDODEMENTIA** A term used to designate the dementia-like symptoms sometimes seen in people who are depressed, who have experienced drug toxicity, or who have other treatable chemical imbalances of the brain. The dementia-like symptoms may improve or disappear with appropriate treatment.

**PSYCHIATRIST** A physician who specializes in the diagnosis and treatment of mental, behavioral, and brain disorders.

**RESPITE CARE** Care that is provided inside or outside of the home to physically or cognitively impaired individuals for the purpose of giving the primary caregiver time off. Respite care is usually purchased through an agency or by private arrangement and can be for varying lengths of time, from a few hours to days or weeks. Some Department of Veterans Affairs Nursing Homes have respite care programs for eligible veterans.

**SPEECH-LANGUAGE PATHOLOGIST** An individual trained to evaluate and treat communication and related disorders. Some speech-language pathologists have special training in evaluating and treating swallowing problems. Most speech-language pathologists have graduate college degrees (MA or Ph.D.) and hold the Certificate of Clinical Competence (CCCSP) granted by the American Speech-Language-Hearing Association. These individuals work in hospitals, clinics, nursing homes, and in private practice as well as in schools and other settings.

**WILL** A written document that stipulates how a person's assets will be distributed after his death.

# Index

AAMI. *See* Age-associated
memory impairment.
Acetylcholine, 27
Activities of daily living
(ADLs), 198
Advocacy, 116–117
Age-associated memory
impairment (AAMI), 10
Aging, Area Agency on, 143
Aging, normal, 6–7
Alcohol Abuse Hotline, 186
Alcohol and dementia, 20
Alone, patient living, 69–70
Aluminum, 27–28
Alzheimer's Association, 107,
111, 118, 137, 143, 179
Alzheimer's disease
alcohol and, 119
aluminum, role in, 27–28
alone, patient living, 69–70
assets of patient, 131–132
behavior changes in, 23–24
behavior, problem, 149–175
(*see also* Behaviors,
problem)
books about, 187–194
caffeine and, 119
causes of, 27–28
children and, 105–107
church resources, 112
communication in, 26–27,
31–37, 39–43, 45–47 (*see
also* Communication)
comprehension problems in, 33
conversation, maintenance
of, 42
DAT (Dementia of the
Alzheimer's Type), 18
day care for, 112–113
defined, 198
decline rates in, 21, 35–36
depression in, 23

Alzheimer's disease *(continued)*
diagnosis of, 17–18
digression in, 33–34
discomfort, signs of, 92–93
early, 7–14, 31–37, 59–72
evaluation of, 36–37
expectations, realistic, 124
expenses of patient, 132
family, communicating with,
95–107
friends, communicating with,
95–107
financial advisors and, 127–138
government agencies and,
139–148
group involvement in, 68
guardianship and, 130
health care professionals and,
115–125
health insurance, 128
hearing loss and, 56
inconsistent patterns in, 25
incontinence in, 26, 46
informing patient of disease,
67–68
language functions in, 12–13
legal advisors and, 127–138
medications and, 119, 121–122
memory changes in, 7–12, 22,
60–62
middle stages of, 39–43, 73–86
neuropsychologist, 36–37
nursing homes, 179
organizations helping with,
182–186
personality and, 13–14, 22–23
physical appearance in, 25–26
physical functioning in, 26
power of attorney and, 129–130
pragmatics, 47
private service agencies and,
139–148